Men's Hairdressing

Hairdressing And Beauty Industry Authority Series – related titles

Hairdressing

Mahogany Hairdressing: Steps to Cutting, Colouring and Finishing Hair
Martin Gannon and Richard Thompson

Mahogany Hairdressing: Advanced Looks   Richard Thompson and Martin Gannon

Essensuals, Next Generation Toni & Guy: Step by Step

Professional Men's Hairdressing   Guy Kemer and Jacki Wadeson

The Art of Dressing Long Hair   Guy Kemer and Jacki Wadeson

Patrick Cameron: Dressing Long Hair   Patrick Cameron and Jacki Wadeson

Patrick Cameron: Dressing Long Hair Book 2   Patrick Cameron

Bridal Hair   Pat Dixon and Jacki Wadeson

Trevor Sorbie: Visions in Hair   Kris Sorbie and Jacki Wadeson

The Total Look: The Style Guide for Hair and Make-up Professionals   Ian Mistlin

Art of Hair Colouring   David Adams and Jacki Wadeson

Start Hairdressing: The Official Guide to Level 1   Martin Green and Leo Palladino

Hairdressing – The Foundations: The Official Guide to Level 2   Leo Palladino

Professional Hairdressing: The Official Guide to Level 3
Martin Green, Lesley Kimber and Leo Palladino

Men's Hairdressing: Traditional and Modern Barbering   Maurice Lister

African-Caribbean Hairdressing   Sandra Gittens

The World of Hair: A Scientific Companion   Dr John Gray

Salon Management   Martin Green

Beauty Therapy

Beauty Therapy – The Foundations: The Official Guide to Level 2
Lorraine Nordmann

Professional Beauty Therapy: The Official Guide to Level 3
Lorraine Nordmann, Lorraine Appleyard and Pamela Linforth

Aromatherapy for the Beauty Therapist   Valerie Ann Worwood

Indian Head Massage   Muriel Burnham-Airey and Adele O'Keefe

The Official Guide to Body Massage   Adele O'Keefe

An Holistic Guide to Anatomy and Physiology   Tina Parsons

The Encyclopedia of Nails   Jacqui Jefford and Anne Swain

Nail Artistry   Jacqui Jefford, Sue Marsh and Anne Swain

The Complete Nail Technician   Marian Newman

The World of Skin Care: A Scientific Companion   Dr John Gray

Safety in the Salon   Elaine Almond

Men's Hairdressing
Traditional and Modern Barbering

Second Edition

Maurice Lister

THOMSON

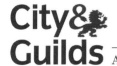

Australia • Canada • Mexico • Singapore • Spain • United Kingdom • United States

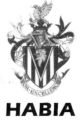

HABIA

THOMSON

Men's Hairdressing: Traditional and Modern Barbering
Second Edition

Copyright © Thomson Learning 2004

The Thomson logo is a registered trademark used herein under licence.

City & Guilds name and logo are the registered trade marks of the City and Guilds of London Institute and are used under licence.

For more information, contact Thomson Learning, High Holborn House, 50–51 Bedford Row, London WC1R 4LR or visit us on the World Wide Web at: http://www.thomsonlearning.co.uk

British Library Cataloguing-in-Publication Data
A catalogue record for this book is available from the British Library

ISBN 1-86152-916-3

First edition published 2000 by Macmillan Press Ltd
Reprinted 2001 by Thomson Learning
Reprinted 2002 by Thomson
This edition published by Thomson Learning 2004
Reprinted 2005 by Thomson Learning

Typeset by Meridian Colour Repro Ltd, Pangbourne-on-Thames, Berkshire

Printed in Croatia by Zrinski d.d.

347068

Contents

Level 3 Advanced menswork

Foreword

I can remember the furore when we first started developing occupational standards for hairdressing over whether men's and ladies' hairdressing should be combined or left separate for the NVQs that were being launched in 1989. The result was that men's hairdressing was combined into the NVQ Level 2 in Hairdressing and for many a year there was a vocal and passionate plea for a separate qualification. In 1999 when the first edition of Maurice's book came out I wrote that this book would serve to develop the talent that exists in men's hairdressing.

In only four years we have seen more and more top hairdressers producing superb images of fascinating styles and quirky cuts. There is a rich vein of talent in men's hairdressing in the UK and I'm convinced that Maurice's commitment to education and his passionate belief in his work are instrumental in this growth. In 2003 HABIA launched the new barbering standards that are now available as NVQ/SVQs.

Maurice believes in the future of men's hairdressing. I do too. Read this book and you will join us.

Alan Goldsbro
Chief Executive Officer
HABIA

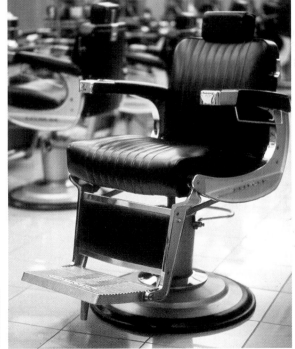

Vidal Sassoon

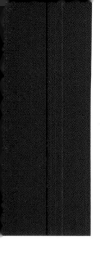

Acknowledgements

On a personal note, I would like to thank my wife, Dawn, Lib Wright, Marie Taylor, Development Editor Jim Collins, Emily Ferguson and all at the publisher, and all at the Hairdressing and Beauty Industry Authority for their patience, encouragement and support.

The author and publishers would like to thank the following for providing pictures for the book: Vidal Sassoon, Nigel Sillis, Guillaume Vappereau, Jacki Wadeson, Guy Kremer, Dr John Gray (Procter & Gamble), Redken, Wella, Dr A.L. Wright (Consultant Dermatologist, Bradford Royal Infirmary), Dr M.H. Beck (Consultant Dermatologist, Salford Royal Hospital), S. Lewis, Martin Turner, Helena Royle (Regis International Ltd), L'Oréal, Salon Ambience, Saks: Premier Collection, Claudia Woolley, Hair and Beauty Industry Authority, City & Guilds, Forfex Professional, Exit Hairdressing, Patrick Cameron, Charlie Miller, Simon Shaw, WAHL, Lee Stafford, MK Hair Studio, Daniel Hill, Charles Worthington, Ralph Kleeli, Goldwell Professional Haircare, Fudge, Comby, Sharon Brigden – SLB Communications, BaByliss Pro, Olymp, Regis International Ltd, Patricia Livingston, Paul Stafford, Clynol, David Adams, John J. Dibbons, Joico, Sorisa, Depilex, Chris Foster, Joshua Lomotey (Soft Sheen Carson), Sandra Gittens, Thornton Howdle Photography, Chris Mullen – Flanigans, Adam Young, Steven Sullivan & Pekka Ikomi of Diligence – Artistic Hair Design, West Ealing, London (www.diligence.co.uk).

The author and publishers would also like to thank the following: Erik Lander and Simon Shaw, who were involved in some of the various techniques photographs taken for this book; Forfex Professional for sponsoring many of the photos for this new edition; Sheffield College for the loan of a barber's chair; Ian Lea Photography and his assistant, Paul (Spud) Edwards for involvement in many of the step by steps which appear in chapters 4, 5, 6, 10, 11, 12 and 13. Thank you Frontier Medical Products (www.sharpsafe.co.uk) for the image of the sharps container. Special thanks to Barrie Carter for the offer of a photograph of his grandfather's barber's shop and to Nigel Sillis for supplying photographs of his father, Henry Sillis's barber's shop. Thanks also to Christopher Selleck for the offer of photographs of his high-frequency equipment. Thank you Adam Young for providing the facial hair illustrations in Chapter 13, 'Designing facial hair shapes'. With great appreciation to Steven Sullivan and Pekka Ikomi of Diligence Artistic Hair Design for providing the step by steps in the final chapter, 'Design and create patterns in hair'. You should see further examples of their creative and artistic work in their book *Diligence: Volume One* available to view on www.diligence.co.uk or to buy from the Internet site www.superbad.co.uk. With great appreciation to Brendan O'Sullivan and the Regis Artistic Team for supplying the front cover picture and the section opening pages for Level 2 and Level 3 Menswork. Finally, thanks to all those kind people who have allowed us to use photographs of their hair.

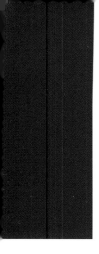

Introduction

Although men make up about 50 per cent of the population, traditionally few hairdressers have specialised in the barbering skills required to develop the men's business. Indeed, some traditional barbering skills were in danger of being lost. Increasing interest in male grooming has provided additional business opportunities for the skilled barber and has, along with the frequent use of barbering techniques in women's hairdressing, further increased the demand for barbering skills.

I originally wrote this book both to help address this demand and to help ensure that the traditional skills are not lost. I am, therefore, delighted that this new edition now covers the 'Menswork' that for the first time is recognised in the new Barbering NVQs/SVQs at Levels 2 and 3 and City & Guilds Specialist Awards and Barbering Diploma. Whether you are an experienced hairdresser or just starting out on your career, the book provides you with all the information necessary to help you develop your potential in barbering. For those undertaking the awards I have included revision questions to help you prepare for examinations. For experienced barbers, I have also included information to help you consolidate your knowledge and skills, which I hope will in turn provide inspiration to develop new services and increase the men's business.

I hope you enjoy reading the book as much as I have enjoyed writing it!

Maurice Lister

NVQ/SVQ Units — Chapters	G1	G5	G6	G7	G8	G9	H2	H8	H9	H12	H13	H14	H17	H18	H19	H20	H21	H22	H24	H29	H30	H34
1 Barbering – origins		✓#	✓#		✓#																	
2 Client care for men	✓*	✓	✓	✓	✓*	✓																
3 Shampooing and conditioning men's hair	✓*				✓*				✓													
4 Cutting facial hair using basic techniques	✓*				✓*			✓														
5 Cutting men's hair using basic techniques	✓*				✓*		✓						✓*									
6 Drying and finishing men's hair	✓*				✓*							✓	✓*									
7 Colouring men's hair	✓*		✓#		✓*						✓#								✓*		✓#	
8 Perming men's hair	✓*		✓#		✓*					✓#									✓*	✓#		
9 Scalp massage	✓*				✓*									✓								
10 Advanced men's hair cutting	✓*				✓*												✓		✓*			
11 Shaving	✓*		✓#		✓*										✓							
12 Face massage	✓*		✓#		✓*																	✓
13 Designing facial hair shapes	✓*				✓*											✓			✓*			
14 Design and create patterns in hair	✓*				✓*													✓				

✓ = This chapter fulfills the NVQ/SVQ barbering unit

* = Further aspects relevant to men's hairdressing are covered in the chapter

\# = Some aspects relevant to men's hairdressing are covered in the chapter. For more information, see Palladino, *Hairdressing – The Foundations, Level 2*, 4th ed and Green and Palladino, *Professional Hairdressing – The Official Guide to Level 3*, 4th ed.

Signposting of the Level 2 and Level 3 Barbering NVQ/SVQ units covered in this book

Barbering – from its origins to the present day

1

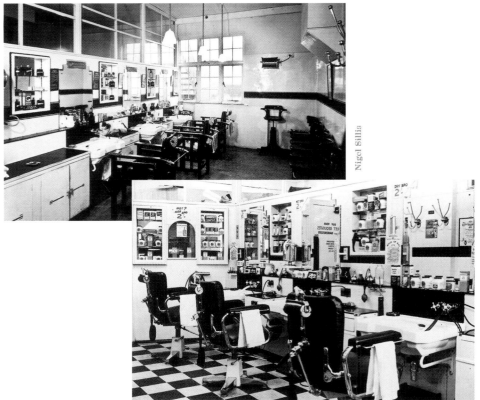

Nigel Sillis

Nigel Sillis

Learning objectives

Barbering has a long and varied past which should be considered by anyone who has an interest in the work of the barber.

This chapter discusses the evolution of barbering to the present day and covers the following topics:

- the origins of barbering
- the meaning of the word 'barber'
- barbering in the ancient world
- the significance of 'barber-surgeons'
- the origin and meaning of the barber's pole
- unusual barber's shop services
- the development of barbering techniques to the present day

The origins of barbering

Barbering may accurately be described as one of the oldest professions in the world. Archaeologists have found simple cutting implements made from sharpened flints and bones, which show that haircutting was practised as long ago as 30,000 years BC. The Egyptians were the first to develop techniques and tools that we might recognise in hairdressing today. Excavation of Egyptian pyramids has unearthed many combs and cutting tools, including razors made of tempered copper and bronze that were used by Egyptians nearly 6000 years ago.

The word 'barber' derives from the Latin word *barba*, meaning 'beard'. Many barbering skills developed because of the importance of the beard in past times. A beard was often considered to be a sign of wisdom and strength and, not surprisingly, also of manhood. The beard has been important in many religions throughout the ages and in some is still important today.

Barbering in ancient times

Organised barbering services were offered as long ago as 1500BC. In ancient Egypt many men had their beard and their head shaved. Egyptian barbers often preferred to work outdoors, because of the hot climate. The barber would meet his clients in the street, where the client would kneel while the barber casually went about his work in full view of passers by.

Although popular in ancient Egypt, shaving did not become commonplace in most other countries until around 400BC, by which time hairstyling and barbering had evolved into highly developed crafts.

In ancient Greece wealthy men regularly had their hair cut and styled, often by their servants, but most members of the poorer classes still wore long hair and beards. In about 335BC Alexander the Great, ruler of Greece at the time, promoted widespread shaving when he ordered his army to remove their beards. This was a strategy to overcome his enemies' tactic of grasping the Greek soldiers' beards during battle. Alexander himself was clean-shaven, which was unusual at that time, when most rulers wore beards, and this too encouraged shaving as men who admired him copied his example.

In Rome by about 300BC barbering services had become available to the general population. Slaves were still forced to wear their beards and hair long, as a sign of their lower status, but most other men visited the barber's shop. Roman men were usually clean-shaven so the barbers' shops were much frequented. They were used as meeting places, and were known to be good places to catch up with the local gossip. Many Roman barbers enjoyed considerable wealth and status in Roman society because of the success of these early shops.

Barber-surgeons

By the Middle Ages barbering services were well established in England and across most of Europe, but barbers were no longer only shaving and haircutting. These early barbers were also the pioneers of many medical treatments. Because they performed both barbering and surgery, they were known as barber-surgeons. They frequently carried out bloodletting and simple surgery, and also pulled teeth – a simple form of dentistry.

The barber's pole

The familiar red-and-white striped barber's pole originated as the symbol of the barber-surgeons and their work in bloodletting. Bloodletting involved cutting a vein on the patient's arm, in order to let out 'bad blood'. Many ailments were thought to be caused by 'bad blood', which was sometimes said to have been affected by evil spirits. Although it was widely believed that removing this blood would bring about a speedy recovery, this treatment is not known to have been very successful. On the contrary, infection would often develop at the site of the cut and this would lead to other serious illnesses.

Wounds were dressed with cloth bandages. In those days the bandages were used over and over again: although they were white at first, with repeated use they became stained. Whilst hanging outside the barbers' shop to dry, they would twist together with new white bandages, forming the red-and-white striped pattern familiar to us now as the barber's pole.

Some barbers' poles also have a blue stripe, and a small bowl hanging beneath. In this instance the pole is said to represent the post that the patient held onto whilst undergoing treatment. The blue stripe represents the blood from the veins, the red stripe the blood from the arteries. The arteries should not have been cut at all, but sometimes they were, by mistake; this illustrates how hazardous the treatment was. The bowl hanging beneath is often said to represent the bowl used to collect the patient's blood. In reality, it is more likely to have been the bowl used to collect lather during shaving.

A barber's pole

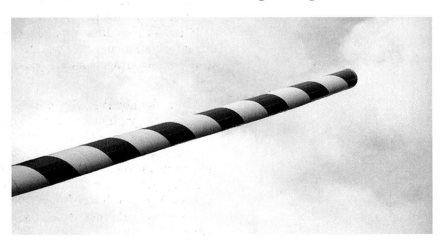

During the 13th century the 'Barbers Company of London' was established, to help regulate and protect the developing barbering profession. Within a few years some of the barber-surgeons began to favour surgery and formed a 'Surgeons' Company' or 'Guild'. In the middle of the 1500s, after many years of disagreement, Henry VIII of England created an Act that united barbers and surgeons under one corporation. Under this Act barbers were prohibited from performing surgery, although they could continue bloodletting and teeth pulling; and the surgeons were prohibited from performing barbering and shaving services.

The barber and surgeon had been united in one profession for over 500 years when they were finally separated in 1745. George II of England passed an Act that divided barbers and surgeons into two distinct corporations. The 'Worshipful Company of Barbers' was formed and barbers dropped their use of the name 'barber-surgeons'. Since then barbers have not performed any medical services, but in many high streets today you will still see the red-and-white striped pole as a symbol of barbers' long, varied and significant past.

Unusual barber's shop services

In times past barber's also became known for performing other unusual services, such as making and mending umbrellas and singeing.

Singeing involved the barber using either a lighted wax taper or electrical singeing equipment to singe the ends of the hair after cutting (most barbers preferred the wax taper). At the time, singeing was commonly thought to 'stop the hair bleeding', as it was believed that the goodness or life of the hair would run out through the cut open end of the hair shaft, but we now know this is not correct. However, it was found to sometimes help reduce fragilitas crinium (split ends), as the cells that make up the hair were fused together by the heat of the flame or heated appliance and so were less able to split apart. The flame also had antiseptic properties and singeing with this method could be useful in the removal of parasites that attach themselves to the hair. Stray hairs left after cutting could also be removed easily to create a smoother finish, especially on shorter styles.

Singeing services demanded that great care was taken to avoid damage to the hair or the barber or client being burnt. A thorough check was always made before starting the service to ensure that the client was not wearing any flammable hair dressings, such as hairspray, as such substances could quickly ignite and cause serious harm. The barber, too, had to ensure he was not wearing such dressings on his hair. Other flammable substances were also kept well clear of the area during the service, e.g. hairspray could not be used by an adjacent barber.

The singeing process resembled the sectioning system used in cutting. At the end of the haircut the barber would retake the sections of hair as in cutting a uniform layer, e.g. at 90° to the head. A tail comb or sometimes the bottom of the taper was used to lift the section, which was transferred to and held in the other hand

Singeing – twisted method

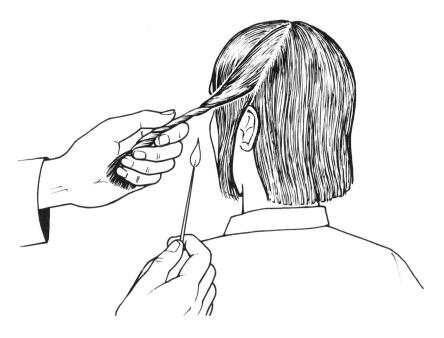

Singeing – flat method

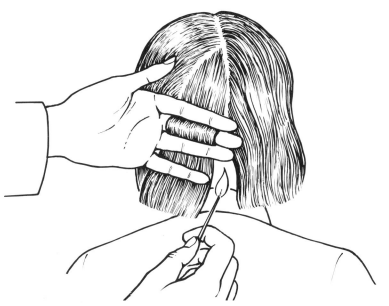

whilst the flame would be quickly run along the ends of the hair. This was continued around the head and when completed the hair would be dressed and finished with products, as required by the client. On longer hair, stray or frayed hairs further up the hair shaft were removed by either a twisting or a flat method.

Singeing has also been used in barber's shops to remove hair growing in the clients' noses and on their ears, as the flame could quickly reach inside these areas. In some countries, e.g. Turkey, barbers can still be seen using singeing for this purpose, but in most barber's shops singeing with a lighted taper is no longer performed because of the risks involved. Over the past few years electrically heated scissors have become available to allow some of the benefits of singeing to be obtained without the need to use an open flame. The scissors are insulated except for their cutting edges in order to protect the client's and barber's skin, and a computer is used to maintain the correct temperature for different hair thicknesses.

Barbering today

Today the term barbering is usually used to describe the work carried out by men's hairdressers, gents' hairdressers, and men's hair stylists – all of whom might be described more simply as 'barbers'.

Of necessity there are many similarities between the work of men's hairdressers and women's hairdressers, but differences do remain between the work each carries out and by their use of different techniques. At one time it was very fashionable to have unisex salons, where both men and women could have their hair cut and styled. Unisex salons used barbering techniques but often did not specialise in men's hairdressing. A barber is someone who specialises in men's hairdressing, and who has developed high-level skills in using barbering techniques, especially for haircutting. These techniques are particularly suitable for dealing with men's hair and for creating men's hairstyles and beard and moustache shapes.

More recently, interest in male grooming has increased, as can be seen from the number of hair and skin-care products now available that are produced specifically for men. Many more men are wearing

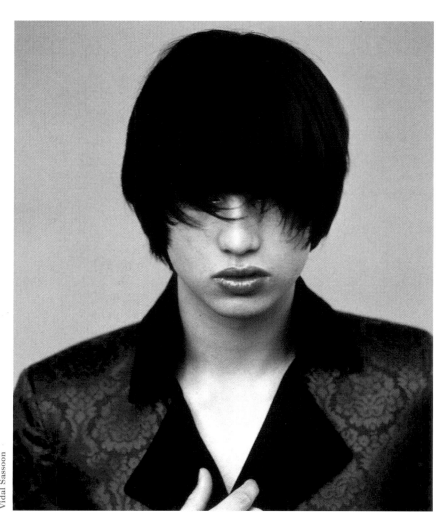

Vidal Sassoon

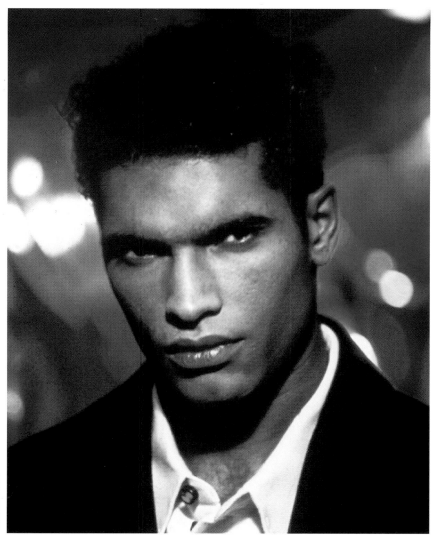

Vidal Sassoon

fashion haircuts and there has been a marked increase in the popularity of beards and moustaches, particularly with young men. This interest has led to many more barbers' shops opening and to an increase in the different services available to men. Today the barber has to be highly skilled and creative in most aspects of hairdressing if he is to meet the needs of his clients and create the varied range of styles that are required. As will become evident through this book, modern men's hairdressing is not just about a 'dry trim' or a 'short back and sides'!

Activity

Visit local barber's shops and use the Internet to research the different types of barber's shops that operate in different places. Find out if their decor and image is traditional or modern and which services are offered. Work out whether their location affects the image and services they offer.

Check your knowledge

1 Describe the origin and meaning of the word 'barber'.

2 Which civilisation developed the first organised hairdressing tools and techniques?

3 Describe the earliest known haircutting tools.

4 How did Alexander the Great influence men's styling at the time?

5 Describe the main services offered by barber-surgeons.

6 Outline the meaning of the striped pattern on the barber's pole.

7 Describe the main benefits of singeing.

8 What unusual service offered by some barber's shops related to the weather?

9 Describe the key differences between a unisex salon and a barber's shop.

10 What have more young men been wearing over recent years?

Client care for men

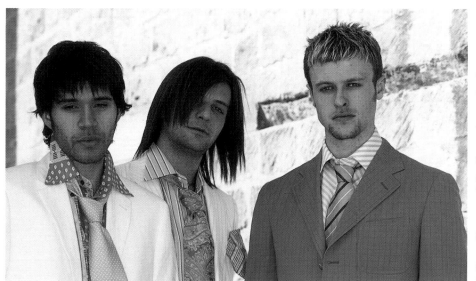

2

Guillaume Vappereau @ Guy Kremer International

Learning objectives

Client care is an essential part of any hairdressing service: it forms an important part of all barbers' work. Providing care involves you working to meet your clients' needs, so that they are satisfied with every aspect of the service you offer. Good client care is a sign of professional standards of work, which all clients should be able to expect.

Client care is achieved through many different skills, including good communication, technical ability, and good manners. The following are some of the important topics covered in this chapter:

- **communicating with your client**
- **recognising the needs of your client**
- **preparing your client for different services**
- **referring your client to others**
- **caring for your client**
- **offering after-care advice**
- **knowing about the hair and the skin**
- **identifying hair and skin conditions and disorders**
- **determining when services should or should not be carried out**
- **salon hygiene**

Client care for men

In essence, client care is the process of caring for your client, and it is the same for both men and women. It involves you looking after your client, ensuring that he is comfortable and safe throughout the service, and that ultimately he is satisfied with the end result.

Client care should begin when the client makes his appointment, which may be in person or over the telephone. It resumes when he enters the salon, and continues until he leaves. Client care should also feature in the offer of after-care advice. This involves you providing advice on after-care products and tips on grooming and styling to help the client maintain his style at home.

In the salon, the first, and essential, stage of client care is the consultation. This must take place before any service is carried out, both for new and existing clients.

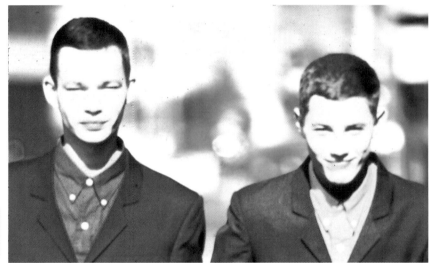

Vidal Sassoon

Consultation

Tip

Sometimes your client may have no idea of what he wants – you will need to use your professional knowledge to guide him. This is an opportunity to develop a good relationship and to establish a loyal client!

Consultation is a two-way process between you and your client, whereby you identify the client's wishes, determine his suitability for the requested service, and provide advice on the most suitable course of action. It involves you both talking to the client and listening to him, so that you can accurately establish his needs. You will need to exchange ideas, and you may need to refer to photographs or sketches to help you clarify the ideas and reach an agreement.

A consultation is *always* necessary

In the barber's shop clients sometimes have their hair cut dry. Indeed, you have probably heard the request 'A dry trim, please' on many occasions. It may seem as if consultation is unnecessary for such clients, especially if they are regular customers at your salon.

However, you must *always* carry out a consultation. This is an opportunity for you to find out about any problems the client has had with his hair which you could help correct. Many clients who change salons say it was because the new barber took the time to find out what they wanted, whereas the previous barber assumed he knew! But more importantly, it is vital that you identify any possible infections or infestations, so that you can protect your other clients, your colleagues and yourself.

Talking with the client

Listen carefully to what your client says – after all, most clients usually know a lot about their own hair. Sometimes you may realise that a satisfactory result would not be likely: you will then need to advise your client to have a different service or a different style from the one he has requested. Remember to do this tactfully, and explain in simple and clear language the reasons for your recommendation.

As part of the consultation, you will need to examine the hair and scalp. The hair should always be *dry* when you do this, so that you can see any problems clearly. Proceed with the service only when you have accurately established what is to be done and have obtained the client's understanding and agreement.

Here are some important points to remember about consultation:

- be tactful
- observe the client's confidentiality at all times
- accurately determine the client's wishes, both before and during the service
- use your skills of questioning and observation to gather all available information
- where necessary, perform tests to determine what services can be carried out: ensure throughout that you work safely and protect the client from harm
- ensure that you identify any adverse conditions of the hair or skin – if you suspect that an infection or infestation is present, you must not carry out the service
- before proceeding, ensure that the client understands and agrees with the service
- take into account any hairpieces that the client may be wearing – determine how these may affect the services to be provided
- record information about the client accurately, so that you can retrieve and review it easily on his subsequent visits to the salon

Referring your client to others

Sometimes it is necessary to refer your client on to other specialists who are better able to deal with their particular requirements. Some examples of the conditions that should be referred and which specialists are appropriate are provided in the tables later in this chapter. At other times you may need to seek advice from specialists before you can carry out the service requested. There are several different types of internal and external specialist advice available, relevant to the conditions you are likely to see when providing hairdressing services. It is important that you know what each specialist does and how they may be contacted. Here are some examples of the specialists and their areas of advice or work that are most often referred to in hairdressing salons.

Health & Safety

Remember – if you are in doubt about conditions or disorders on a client always seek advice before commencing the service, especially if you suspect a condition may be infectious. Make sure that you know and follow your salon's policy for referring clients on to others.

Specialist	*Area of advice/work*	*Contact details*
● Senior, experienced colleagues, e.g. those with Barbering or Hairdressing N/SVQ Level 3 ● Salon manager	● Clarification of simple recognisable conditions and disorders seen within the salon ● Second technical opinion and advice on service requirements ● Confirmation of the need to refer clients on to external specialists	● Your salon should have a communication policy that sets out who you refer to in the salon with these types of problems
● Manufacturers' information and advice lines	● Some general hair care advice ● Usually more specific advice about using the manufacturer's own products	● Telephone numbers, postal address and online address usually shown on products ● Details also in telephone directories
● General Practitioner (GP) or Doctor ● Trichologist (Clinical Trichology)	● General medicine ● Diseases and disorders of the hair and scalp	● Clients should contact their own GP ● Local telephone directories ● Institute of Trichologists www.trichologists.org.uk
● Dermatologist	● Skin diseases and disorders	● Referral usually through the client's own GP
● NHS Direct UK	● General medical advice within the UK over the telephone or online	● 0845 4647 ● www.nhsdirect.nhs.uk
● Chemist (Pharmacist)	● General health advice and the provision of medicines and treatments	● Local pharmacy details found in regional telephone directories

Caring for your client

Tip

Never carry out a hairdressing service without a consultation. It is unprofessional and is likely to result in a dissatisfied client, or worse!

Tip

Make sure you make a record of any staining or damage to the client's clothes and inform your manager or supervisor.

Throughout the service, you must take care of your client and ensure that he is comfortable. This can be achieved by following some simple rules:

- **Security** Ensure that the client's coat and belongings are placed safely in the place specified by your salon.
- **Preparation** Gather together all the materials, products, tools and equipment you will require before you begin work.
- **Comfort** Ensure that the protective gown, the cutting collar, towels, cottonwool pads and so on all remain in their correct places before and during services. During cutting services, remove excess hair cuttings from the client and the gown or cutting collar.
- **Reading and refreshments** In accordance with your salon's policy, offer the client reading materials or refreshments, especially during lengthy processes such as colouring and perming.
- **Explanation** As the service progresses, let the client know what you are doing – especially during perming, colouring or lightening. Explain how long the service might take, ask the client if he has any questions, and reassure him if necessary.
- **Finishing** Ensure that the client's clothes are not damp or stained, and that all loose hair clippings have been removed. Return the client's coat and belongings to him. Offer to make the next appointment for him.

Preparing the client

Gowning and protecting the client

Following the consultation, and before you proceed with the services to be carried out, the client must be correctly gowned and protected. Which gowns, towels and so on are needed will depend on the service to be performed: this is explained in more detail in the relevant chapters. Here are some *general* rules to follow when gowning and protecting clients.

Tip

Remember to lock chairs that swivel so that they will not spin around whilst the clients are sitting down.

- **The chair** Before seating the client, check that the chair is clean: remove any hairs that may have fallen on the seat or the back of the chair. Position the chair and the client in the correct position for the service to be carried out.
- **The gown** Place a tissue or neck strip around the client's collar, then secure a clean gown into position.
- **Shampoos** If the client is to be shampooed, one or two towels will be required. For a back-wash basin, one towel should be placed over the back and shoulders. For a front-wash basin, one towel should be placed across his chest and

Basic gowning

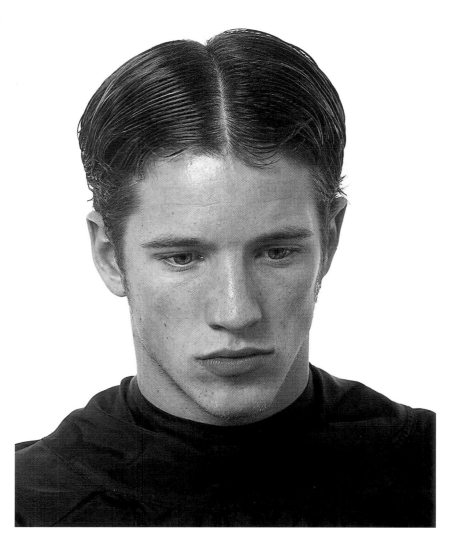

tucked in at the neck, and a second towel placed over the shoulders and the first towel.

- **Cutting** If cutting, use a cutting collar and/or cutting cape. Make sure no hair can fall down between the client and the chair back.
- **Shaving** When shaving, place a clean towel around the front of the client. A paper towel should then be placed over the towel and across the client's shoulder (from his neck towards your body).

Preparing the client's hair

The client's hair must be freed from any tangles before you can work with it effectively.

1   Begin by teasing the hair apart with your fingers. If the hair is long and very tangled, follow these simple steps.

2   Using a wide-toothed comb and beginning near the nape, take a section of hair and comb through the ends, removing any

Client gowned for hair cutting

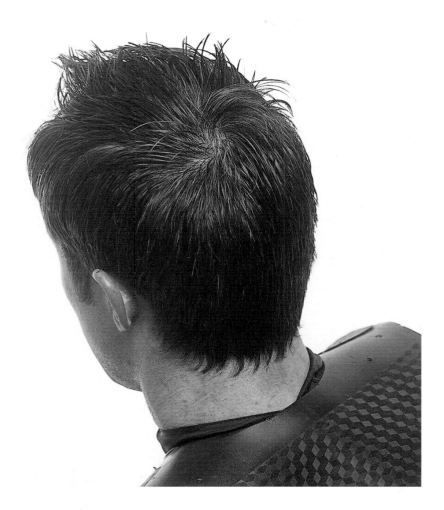

tangles. Gradually work up the section of hair until the comb will travel easily from the roots to the ends.

3   Continue taking sections in this way, working up the back and sides, until all the tangles are removed. Take care not to jerk the client's head whilst combing the hair.

After-care advice

You should provide advice on after-care products, and tips on grooming and styling to help your client maintain his hair at home. This is also an opportunity for you to suggest other beneficial salon services.

Here are some suggestions for you to consider:

- always offer advice and tips on styling to clients who have had new styles
- encourage clients to ask about services
- suggest products that will benefit clients most and keep their hair in good condition.

The structure of the hair and skin

Anyone with an interest in providing hairdressing services must understand the basic properties of the hair and the skin, and the effects that certain services have on their structures. The location and function of the cuticles, cortex, hair follicles and blood supply must all be understood, as these often affect the choice of techniques and how they are applied. The different types of hair, the hair-growth cycle and the hair's chemical composition and physical properties should also be known.

The hair

Hairs are to be found covering all parts of the body, except for the palms of the hands, the soles of the feet and the eyelids.

Types of hair

There are three different types of hair.

Lanugo hair

Lanugo hair is a very fine downy hair that covers the body of unborn and newborn babies. It is usually lost either at birth or soon afterwards.

Vellus hair

Vellus hair is very fine hair which occurs on most parts of the body. It can often be seen on the cheeks of women, and on the forehead

Vellus hair

Dr John Gray

and scalp of men with male-pattern alopecia (baldness), as the vellus hair is not usually lost.

Terminal hair

Terminal hair is the longer hair that occurs on the head, arms, legs, eyebrows and pubic areas, and on the face and chest in men.

Hair structure

Each individual hair shaft consists of three layers.

The cuticle

The cuticle is the thin outer layer of the hair shaft, which is made up of colourless cells. The cells look like scales and overlap like tiles on a roof. The scales point *away* from the roots and *towards* the ends: the hair feels smooth if you rub your hand from the roots to the ends, but rough if you rub it from ends to the roots, especially if the cuticles are damaged.

The cuticle forms a protective surface to the hair and so helps to maintain its condition. Healthy hair shines because all the cuticle cells are lying flat and the light is reflected. Damaged and rough cuticles trap the light, making the hair appear dull and lifeless.

Hair cuticles, seen under an electron microscope

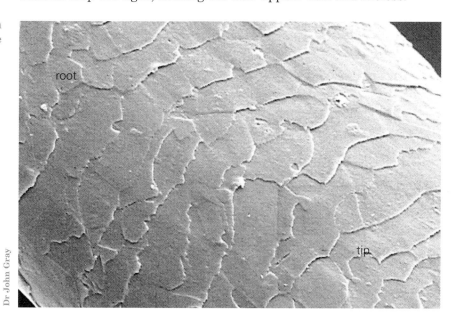

Dr John Gray

The cortex

The cortex is the middle layer of the hair. It is by far the largest part of the hair and is the main source of the hair's strength. The cortex is where the changes take place during blow-drying, perming, relaxing, lightening and colouring.

The cortex is made up of many long strands of fibres, which resemble springs twisted together. The largest strands are the cortical cells, which are themselves made of smaller bundles called

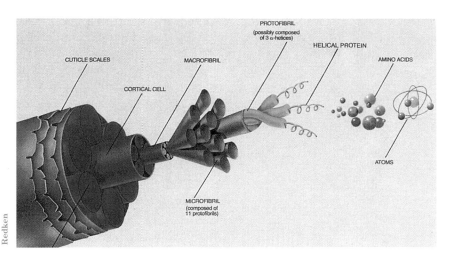

Redken

macrofibrils. These in turn are made up of bundles of microfibrils, and these in turn of bundles of protofibrils. All these fibres and cells are held together by linkages and chains which determine the hair's elasticity, thickness, strength and curl pattern.

The colour of the hair is determined by the pigment, which is also found in the cortex.

The medulla

The medulla is the very fine core of the hair. It does not have any real function and is not always present, particularly in fine blonde hair.

The chemical composition of hair

The cortical cells are made from molecules of amino acids. These are combinations of the elements carbon, oxygen, nitrogen, hydrogen and sulphur.

Amino acids are joined together by peptide bonds, forming long chains called polypeptides. These in turn form proteins.

The principal protein in hair is called keratin, and it is also found in the nails and the skin. Keratin has elastic properties which make the hair flexible and allow it to be stretched and curled without breaking.

Keratin chains are combined in hair in a coiled, spring-like shape. They are held in this shape by linkages *within* chains and *between* chains. There are three different kinds of linkage:

- disulphide bridges or sulphur bonds
- salt links
- hydrogen bonds.

The disulphide bridges are very strong linkages, but they can be broken and remade using chemicals during processes such as perming. It is this breaking and remaking of disulphide bridges that allows hair to be moulded to a new *permanent* shape.

Salt links

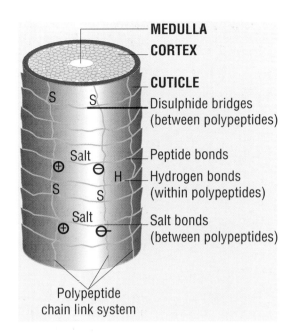

MEDULLA
CORTEX
CUTICLE
Disulphide bridges (between polypeptides)
Peptide bonds
Hydrogen bonds (within polypeptides)
Salt bonds (between polypeptides)

Polypeptide chain link system

The salt links and hydrogen bonds are much weaker, and are easily broken just with water. This allows the hair to be easily stretched and moulded, as when blow-waving. This change is only temporary, however, and the hair will return to its natural state when moisture enters. (See Chapter 6.)

The physical characteristics of hair

Hair is hygroscopic: it absorbs water from the atmosphere. The amount of water absorbed depends upon the humidity of the atmosphere – how dry or damp the *air* is – as well as how dry the *hair* is.

Hair naturally contains some moisture, which lubricates the fibres and allows the hair to stretch and recoil. Hair is also porous: it will absorb water like a sponge soaking up water. (This is called capillary action.)

Damaged hair is far more porous than healthy hair, and loses its natural moisture much more quickly. This is why it is more difficult to stretch and mould dry and damaged hair.

Hair types

There are three different hair types, each of which can be of fine, medium or coarse textures:

- **Caucasian** or **European** hair is mainly straight or lightly waved
- **Black** or **African-Caribbean** hair has tight curls or kinks
- **Mongoloid** or **Asian** hair is usually very straight and coarse.

Cross-sections through hair: left, Mongoloid; centre, Caucasian; right, African-Caribbean

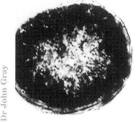
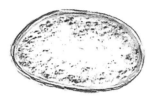
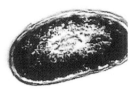

Dr John Gray

Caucasian or European hair

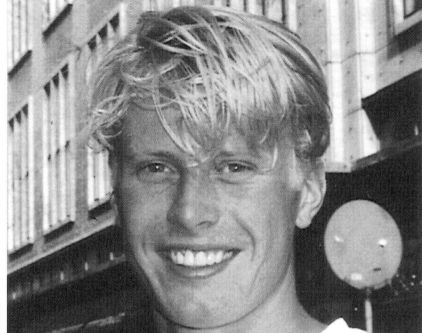

Dr John Gray

Black or African-Caribbean hair

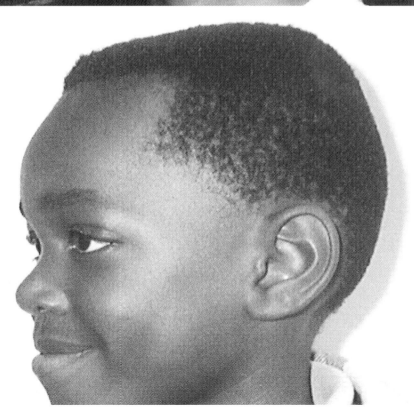

Dr John Gray

Mongoloid or Asian hair

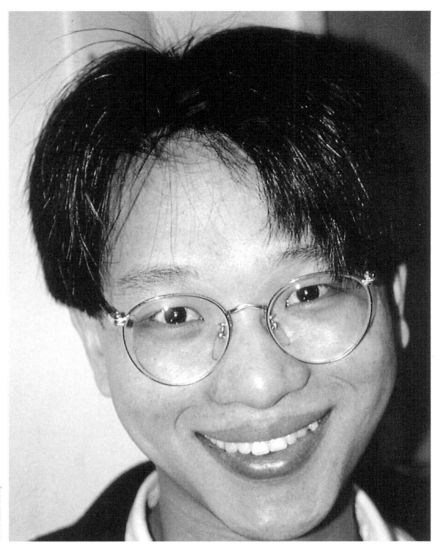

Dr John Gray

Hair growth

Hair grows continually for a period of between about one year and six years. Each individual hair grows following a cycle, which includes a period of growth, rest and loss.

Eventually the hair falls out, but before it leaves the hair follicle (see page 25) a new hair is usually ready to replace it. If a new hair is not present an area of baldness will develop, as in male-pattern baldness. Normally, however, the cycle of growth is not really noticeable: because the hairs are all at different stages of growth, some are always in the growing stage.

Stages of growth

There are three basic stages of growth.

- **Anagen** This is the active growing stage of the hair growth cycle, which may last from about three months to several years.

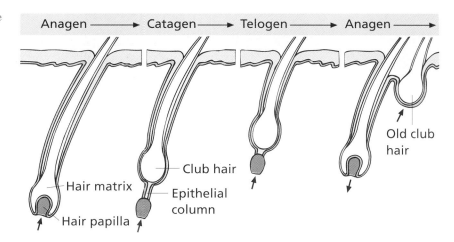

The hair growth cycle

- **Catagen** This is the stage when the hair stops growing. It lasts for about two weeks. During this stage the hair separates from the papilla and begins to move up the follicle.
- **Telogen** This is the resting stage. During this stage the follicle shrinks and separates from the papilla. This stage lasts for only a short period, after which a new anagen stage begins.

Factors affecting hair growth

The healthy growth of new hair can be affected by many different factors. Here are some of the most common and their effects:

- poor health – hair may become thinner, sparse, or stop growing; elasticity, strength and gloss are likely to reduce
- poor diet – as poor health
- increasing age – as poor health
- gender – more men suffer hair loss through male pattern alopecia
- heredity – male pattern alopecia is one type of hereditary condition
- hormones – fluctuating hormone levels affect hair growth rates: male hormones (androgens) speed up hair growth; female hormones (oestrogens) slow it down
- climate and environment – hair may lose elasticity, strength and gloss and may become discoloured
- harsh physical treatment – hair is likely to lose elasticity, strength and gloss; hair breakage likely
- chemicals – overprocessing leads to loss of elasticity, gloss and hair breakage
- disease – some diseases will cause hair loss; others affect growth rates and the composition of the hair.

The skin

The skin is a complex organ which covers the whole of the body. Indeed, it is the largest organ of the body. It has many different layers and it performs several important functions.

Protection

The skin provides a tough, flexible, waterproof covering which protects the underlying tissues from injury. It prevents harmful substances from entering the body unless the skin is cut, and contains a pigment called melanin which absorbs harmful ultraviolet rays from the sun.

The surface of the skin is itself protected by its natural oil, called sebum. This is mildly acidic (about pH 5.6) and has anti-bacterial properties which help prevent the growth of bacteria. Sebum also prevents the loss of water from the underlying layers of the skin, and so prevents the skin from drying out.

Regulation of body temperature

The temperature of the body is regulated through sweating. Sweat evaporates and cools the surface of the skin.

Excretion of waste

Waste products such as water and salt are removed from the body through sweating.

Feeling

The skin contains nerves that allow the sensations of heat, cold, pain and touch to be experienced. These form a warning system that helps us to avoid harm and injury.

Production of vitamin D

When exposed to sunlight, the skin produces vitamin D.

The epidermis

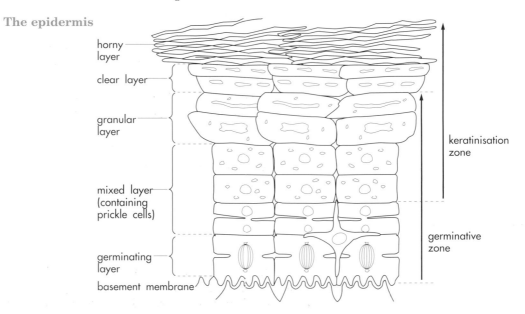

The epidermis

horny layer
clear layer
granular layer
mixed layer (containing prickle cells)
germinating layer
basement membrane

keratinisation zone

germinative zone

The epidermis is the layer of the skin nearest the surface. It is made up of five layers:

- **The horny layer** This forms the outermost part of the skin. It has a hard surface, which is constantly being worn away and renewed by new cells. It takes about one month for cells to move up from the bottom of the epidermis to the top.
- **The clear layer** This is a transparent layer, which contains the protein keratin.
- **The granular layer** This contains granular cells. It is situated between the living cells below and the hardened dead cells above.
- **The mixed layer** This contains a mixture of different live cells, including prickle cells, which lie just below the granular layer. The skin's colour pigment, melanin, is also to be found in this layer.
- **The germinating layer** This lies at the bottom of the epidermis and is connected to the basement membrane, which is attached to the dermis (see below). It is the most active layer, where new epidermal cells are produced.

The dermis

The dermis lies in the middle part of the skin and is much thicker than the epidermis. It has a good supply of blood and is the source of nutrients for the skin.

- **The reticular layer** The lower area of the dermis is composed of protein fibres which allow the skin to expand and contract.
- **The papillary layer** The upper part of the dermis contains tiny projections called papillae, which contain the nerve endings.

The subcutaneous layer

The subcutaneous layer lies below the dermis. It is where the body stores fat.

The hair in skin

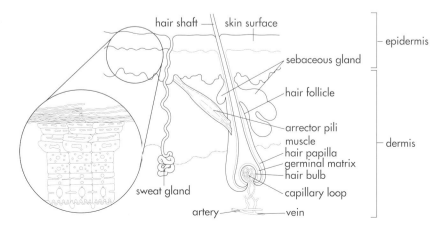

The hair follicle

The hair follicle is the source of the hair's growth. Follicles are found all over the body, except on the lips, the palms of the hands and the soles of the feet.

At the bottom of the follicle is the hair papilla and a tiny group of cells called the germinal matrix. These are supplied with nerves and a good supply of blood to nourish cell growth. Hair is formed when the cells grow and move up the hair follicle. Gradually the cells harden and die, and the hair is formed. First the hair bulb is formed, then more cells are produced, and sooner or later they appear above the skin surface.

The hair papilla and the germinal matrix

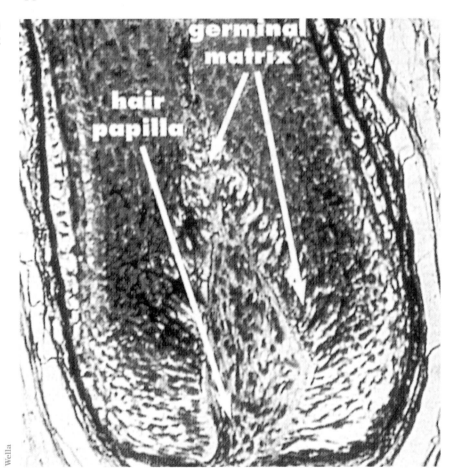

Wella

The sweat gland

The sweat glands are found all over the body. They lie alongside each hair follicle and produce sweat which passes up onto the surface of the skin.

The sebaceous gland

Sebaceous glands or oil glands are found all over the body, except on the palms of the hands and the soles of the feet. They are usually situated alongside the hair follicle, which they open into: this allows their oil, sebum, to be secreted onto the hair and skin.

The arrector pili muscle

The arrector pili muscle is attached at one end to the hair follicle and at the other to the epidermis: when the muscle contracts, the hair stands erect. Together the erect hairs trap a layer of warm air around the body.

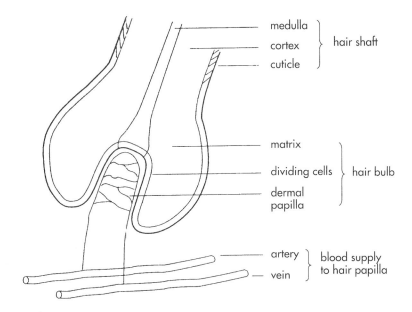

Hair bulb

Conditions of the hair and skin

Bacterial diseases

Condition	Infectious?	Cause	Symptoms	Treatment/ advice
furunculosis (boils and abscesses)	Yes	Infection of the hair follicles by staphylococcal bacteria	Inflamed pus-filled spots with swelling and pain	By a doctor NHS Direct
sycosis barbae (barber's itch)	Yes	A bacterial infection of the hairy parts of the face	Small, yellow spots around the follicle, with irritation and inflammation	By a doctor NHS Direct
impetigo	Yes	A bacterial (staphylococcal or streptococcal) infection of the upper layers of the skin. Sometimes caused by shaving too close, which allows ingrown hairs to develop, which can become infected	Burning irritation with spots appearing, which become dry and crusted. The spots merge to form larger patches	By a doctor NHS Direct
folliculitis (inflammation of the hair follicles)	Yes	A bacterial infection, or sometimes chemical or physical damage	Inflamed follicles	By a doctor NHS Direct

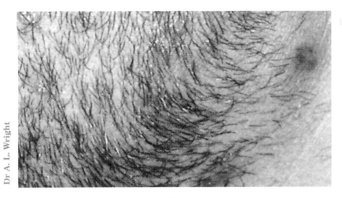

Dr A. L. Wright

Sycosis barbae – barber's itch

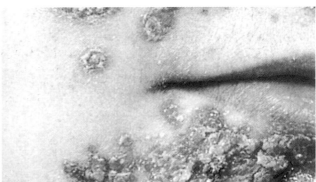

Dr M. H. Beck

Impetigo

Tip

African-Caribbean men can be more susceptible to ingrowing hairs because their tight curly hair more easily grows into the skin. Regular exfoliation to remove the top layers of dead skin cells can help the hair grow out through the follicles and so prevent ingrowing hairs.

Viral diseases

Condition	Infectious?	Cause	Symptoms	Treatment/advice
herpes simplex (cold sore)	Yes	A viral infection of the skin, possibly following exposure to extreme heat or cold, or reaction to food or drugs. The skin may carry the virus for many years	Irritation and swelling with inflammation, followed by the appearance of fluid-filled blisters, usually on and around the lips	By a doctor NHS Direct
warts	Yes	A viral infection at the bottom of the epidermis, which causes the skin to harden and the skin cells to multiply	Raised, roughened skin, often brown or discoloured	By a doctor NHS Direct or products available from a pharmacist

Fungal diseases

Condition	Infectious?	Cause	Symptoms	Treatment/advice
tinea capitis (ringworm of the head)	Yes	A fungal parasite, which infects the skin or hair	Circular areas of greyish white skin, each surrounded by a red ring. The hair is often broken close to the skin and it looks dull	By a doctor NHS Direct

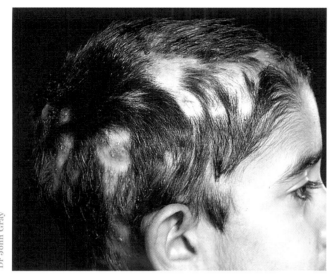

Dr John Gray

Tinea capitis (ringworm)

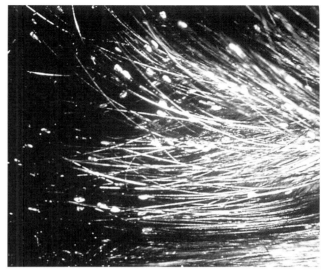

Dr John Gray

Pediculosis capitis

Infestations by parasites (infectious)

Condition	Infectious?	Cause	Symptoms	Treatment/ advice
scabies	Yes	An allergic skin reaction to the presence of the itch mite, a small animal about the size of a pin head, which burrows into the skin, where it lays its eggs	A red rash, usually found in the folds of the skin between the fingers and on the wrists. It is very itchy	By a doctor or with products available from a pharmacist NHS Direct
pediculosis capitis (head lice)	Yes	An infestation of the head by head lice	The lice can be seen by parting the hair, but more commonly the eggs (nits), or the empty egg cases, can be seen stuck to the hairs	By a doctor or with products available from a pharmacist NHS Direct

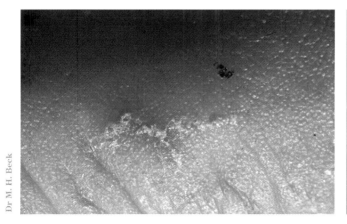

Dr M. H. Beck

Scabies

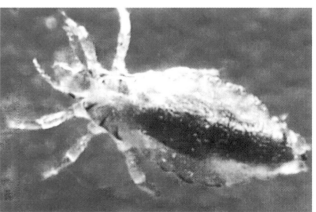

S. Lewis

Pediculosis capitis – head louse

Disorders of the hair and skin

Condition	Infectious?	Cause	Symptoms	Treatment/advice
acne (a condition affecting the hair follicles and sebaceous glands)	No	Not known	Spots or bumps, often seen on the face and forehead, which cause soreness, irritation and inflammation	By a doctor NHS Direct
alopecia (baldness or thin hair growth)	No	The hair follicles are not able to produce new hairs. The causes of alopecia are not fully understood but some forms, such as *alopecia areata*, may be brought on be stress. *Male-pattern alopecia* is hereditary. Pulling, such as when the hair is left in tight plaits for a long period, causes *alopecia traction*. *Cicatrical alopecia* is the result of scarring arising from physical or chemical damage to the follicles	Areas of baldness or thinning hair growth. Male-pattern alopecia often follows the Hamilton pattern	By a doctor or trichologist NHS Direct
canities	No	The colour pigment does not form in new hair growth – often associated with increasing age	White hairs are visible	Tinting

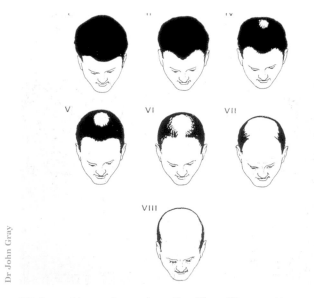

Male-pattern alopecia – the Hamilton pattern

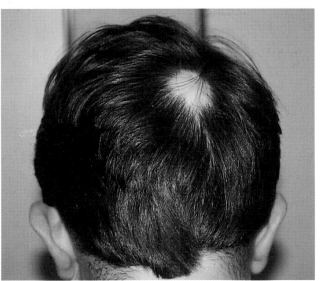

Alopecia areata

Dr John Gray

Dr John Gray

Condition	Infectious?	Cause	Symptoms	Treatment/advice
dandruff (pityriasis capitis)	No	A fungal infection, or through physical or chemical irritation	Small greyish-white flakes of skin	Many anti-dandruff medicines and shampoos are available
eczema and dermatitis	No	Physical irritation or an allergic reaction	The skin may be inflamed and split with weeping areas. There may be some irritation and pain	By a doctor NHS Direct
seborrhoea	No	Over-production of sebum, which may be due to physical or chemical irritants	Greasy, lank hair and greasy skin	Wash regularly using gentle massage movements and warm (not hot) water. A trichologist or doctor should treat extreme cases
psoriasis	No	Unknown	Patches of raised thickened skin, which may be red with silvery or yellow scales. The skin may be sore and/or itchy	By a doctor or a dermatologist NHS Direct

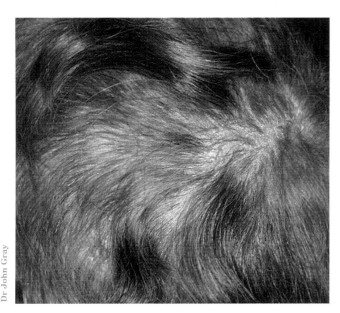

Dr John Gray

Psoriasis

Adverse conditions of the hair and skin

Condition	Infectious?	Cause	Symptoms	Treatment/ advice
fragilitas crinium (split ends)	No	Physical or chemical damage	The ends of the hairs are dry and split	Remove the hair ends by cutting. Use a conditioner
monilethrix (beaded hair)	No	The hair develops irregularly while in the follicle	Bead-like swellings of the hair shafts, which often cause the hair to break close to the skin	By a doctor. Handle with care and use conditioner regularly NHS Direct
trichorrhexis nodosa	No	Physical or chemical damage	Patches of swelling and splitting on the hair shaft	Cutting and conditioning
sebaceous cyst	No	A blocked sebaceous gland	Bumps or lumps, about 10–50mm across, on the scalp or nape	Removal of the cyst by a doctor NHS Direct
damaged cuticle	No	Physical or chemical damage	Rough areas of cuticle. The hair is dry and porous	Apply conditioners, thickeners or restructurants

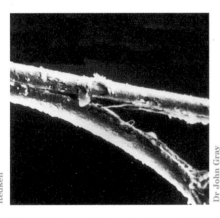

Fragilitas crinium (split ends)

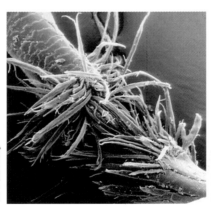

Trichorrhexis nodosa

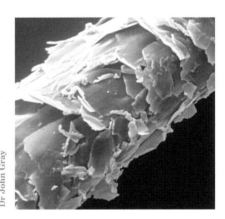

Damaged cuticle

Working safely

The barber must be able to recognise probable infections and infestations of the skin and hair in order to avoid catching them or passing them from one client to another. You must be especially alert to the dangers of two serious conditions that may be contracted through open cuts and abrasions.

AIDS

AIDS stands for acquired immune-deficiency syndrome. It is not a disease but a condition that makes the body more susceptible to diseases, and these may lead to death. To ensure that you protect your clients, your colleagues and yourself, you need to understand how AIDS is transmitted.

AIDS is caused by a virus known as the human immunodeficiency virus (HIV). People may carry the HIV virus – they are said to be 'HIV-positive' – without developing AIDS. However, a person who is HIV-positive could pass the virus to another person – but only if that person's infected body fluids, such as blood, come into contact with the other person's body fluids. Although this occurs most commonly through unprotected sex or when drug addicts share needles, the virus *can* be transferred through a cut or through broken skin.

The virus cannot live for long outside the body – you cannot catch it from toilet seats, for example.

Hepatitis B

Hepatitis B is a disease affecting the liver. This too is caused by a virus, the hepatitis B virus (HBV). HBV is transmitted through infected body fluids such as blood, and also through infected water.

Hepatitis can affect the victim for a long time, and it can be fatal. Treatments are available, but the virus is known to be very resistant. It can survive a long time outside the body, so it is vital that you maintain a high standard of hygiene.

A vaccination is available to protect against hepatitis B. As a barber you are at risk from this virus, so you should consider having this vaccination.

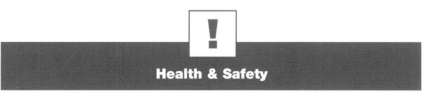

Health & Safety

If you suspect that an infectious condition is present, you must not proceed with the service. Seek advice from your manager or supervisor if necessary, and tactfully suggest that your client go to his doctor.

The clean interior of a modern barber's shop

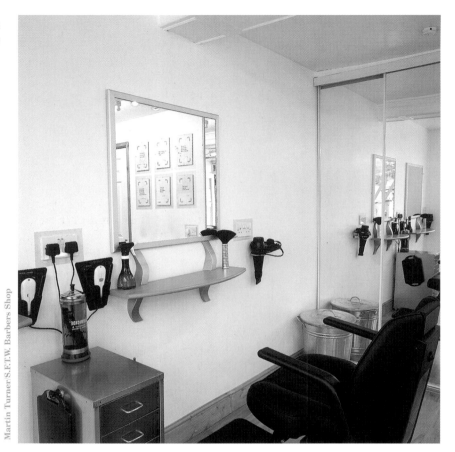

Martin Turner/S.F.T.W. Barbers Shop

Health and safety

The need for hygiene

Effective hygiene is necessary in the salon to prevent infection and cross-infection, which may occur if the salon is dirty or if you or your client has an infectious condition or disease. Cross-infection usually occurs through physical contact with another person or via a tool, such as a razor, which has become infected.

The warm, humid atmosphere in the salon can be the perfect home for infectious organisms. Sterilisation with physical or chemical agents will destroy all the infectious and harmful micro-organisms, however, and sanitation will destroy some but not all micro-organisms. Regular cleaning with bleach or disinfectant will ensure that the risk of infection and cross-infection in the salon is minimised.

General salon hygiene rules

Always follow your salon's health and safety procedures.

- Cover any cuts or open wounds you may have, and ensure they remain covered.
- Maintain a high standard of personal hygiene. Wash your hands regularly.
- Use a clean gown and clean towels for each client.
- Be sure to clean and sterilise tools before using them on clients.
- Keep working surfaces clean. Sanitise them regularly using bleach or disinfectant.
- Store dirty laundry in a sealed container.
- Put waste in suitable bags that can be sealed. Contaminated materials and sharps must be stored and disposed of as specified by the local environmental health authority.

Activities

1 Draw and label a diagram of a hair follicle in the skin.

2 Effective communication is an essential part of the consultation process. Take turns role playing the part of clients who are happy, confused and angry and practice these verbal and non-verbal communication skills with your colleagues:
   - verbal: open questions, probing questions, closed questions
   - non-verbal:
     - written – a telephone message to a client or colleague
     - body language – posture, gestures, nearness and eye contact

   Check your work with your manager or tutor.

3 Visit local chemists and use the Internet to find out what products are available over the counter for treating different conditions of the hair and scalp. Check the prices and compare the products with those in your own salon. Are there any available that you would recommend your manager to keep in stock? Make a list of the products that you stock, noting their key features and benefits. With your manager's permission, share this with your colleagues for use when promoting the products to clients.

4 Part of the barber's role is to sell products and services to clients so that the barber's shop is profitable. Visit the library or use the Internet to research the Consumer and Retail Legislation for promoting and selling products and services. Compare these rules with those in your salon and make a list of the key things that must be adhered to when selling.

5 Practise your selling skills with your colleagues. Make sure that you know your salon's policy for referring clients to other salons or retail outlets when you do not offer requested services or products.

Remember when selling you should:

- look for buying signals – is the client asking about the product or service to show they are interested or changing the subject because they are not?

- provide honest and accurate information about the most suitable product or service for the client:
  - highlight the features – how it works, what it costs
  - highlight the benefits – how it will enhance the client's hair
  - use the product as an aid – let the client handle it, or use pictures to promote the service

- close the sale or offer alternatives:
  - allow the client time to make up his mind – don't push him or you may lose the sale and maybe even the client!
  - confirm the sale when the client is happy with the chosen product or service
  - offer suitable alternatives if the client is unsure
  - if specified by your salon you may refer the client to other salons or outlets if you do not offer the service or product

6 Use the Internet to find out more about bacteria, viruses, fungi and parasites that are the cause of many diseases and disorders. Try to obtain pictures that will help you identify them. Find out how each is contracted and treated. Check your findings with your manager or tutor.

7 Working efficiently so as not to keep clients waiting is an important part of client care. Check your NVQ/SVQ logbook or use the Internet to visit HABIA's website to find out the maximum service times specified for each service offered in barber's shops. Compare these times with the times required by your own salon. Discuss these with your manager to make sure that you understand the reason for any differences.

Check your knowledge

1 State when good client care should begin.
2 Which clients should be consulted before services are carried out?
3 Describe nine points that should be remembered when carrying out a consultation.
4 Outline six rules of caring for your client.
5 What must be removed from the hair before commencing work?
6 State two reasons for providing after-care advice.
7 Describe vellus hair.
8 Describe the middle layer of the hair.
9 Hair is said to be 'hygroscopic'. Describe what this means.
10 When viewed as a cross section, what shape is African-Caribbean hair?

11 Name the hair growth stage where the hair separates from the papilla.

12 List five functions of the skin.

13 Name the two main layers of skin that the hair follicle passes through.

14 Why do we have an arrector pili muscle?

15 Describe the cause and symptoms of sycosis barbae.

16 Describe two different types of infestation that may be seen in a barber's shop.

17 What is meant by the 'Hamilton pattern'?

18 Describe two methods of treatment for fragilitas crinium.

19 Describe how to protect yourself, clients and colleagues from contracting HIV whilst working in the barber's shop.

20 Compare sterilisation with sanitation and outline the key differences.

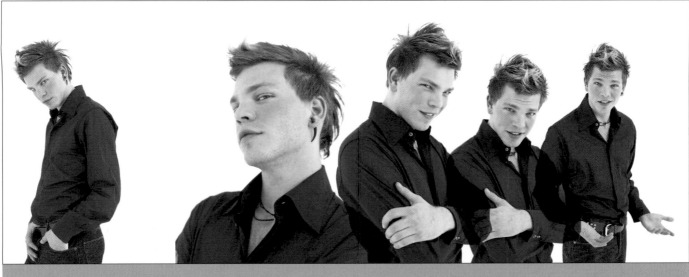

Level 2 Menswork

Shampooing and conditioning men's hair

3

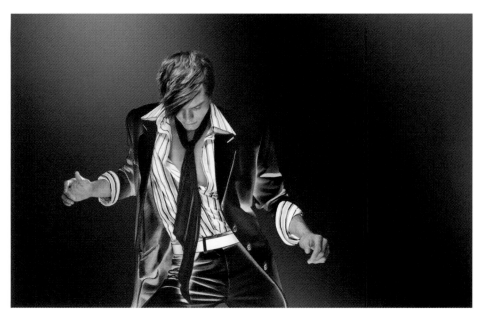

L'Oreal

Learning objectives

The correct use of shampoos and conditioners forms the basis of all good hair care regimes. They help to keep the hair clean and healthy and have an effect on most other hairdressing services. Both at home and in the salon, shampooing and conditioning requires careful thought to make sure that the correct type of product is used. Many different shampoos and conditioners have been developed. The science behind them is not simple, but it must be understood if the barber is to provide accurate services and advice.

In this chapter we will be looking at the techniques used for shampooing and conditioning men's hair and will be covering the following topics:

- **shampooing in the barber's shop**
- **reasons for shampooing and conditioning**
- **how shampoos and conditioners work**
- **selecting the correct product**
- **preparation for shampooing and conditioning**
- **shampooing and conditioning techniques**
- **a shampooing and conditioning procedure**
- **notes on health and safety**

Shampooing in the barber's shop

In the past shampooing and conditioning have been carried out in barber's shops, but the popularity of dry cutting and fact that most men did not have weekly appointments for setting or blow-drying meant that these services were not always used. Dry shampooing, using spirit based lotions or dry powders like talc was also once popular, but these methods are less effective than wet shampooing and are rarely used in barber's shops today.

Many more men now have their hair cut wet and it is shampooed first. Sometimes the hair is shampooed after cutting, particularly on very short haircuts to remove the tiny excess hairs, to make the client feel more comfortable and to obtain the best finish. Other men just enjoy the refreshing and relaxing sensation of the scalp massage provided during shampooing.

The process of shampooing and conditioning is mostly the same for men and women. Some products do differ, usually in their perfume and packaging. Women tend to have hairdressing services that use chemicals more often and so, usually, more women than men need conditioning treatments. One main difference is that in barber's shops the clients often have their hair shampooed at front wash basins rather than at back wash basins. This situation developed mostly because each barber's working station had its own basin installed so that clients did not have to leave the chair to be shampooed.

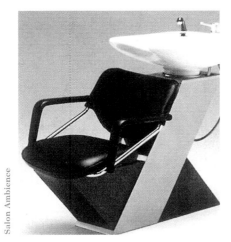

Salon Ambience

Back wash basin

A modern salon

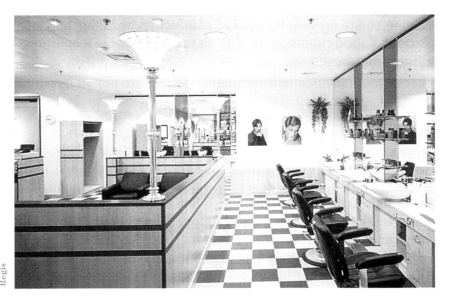

Regis

Reasons for shampooing and conditioning

Shampooing

The main purpose of shampooing is to clean the hair and scalp. A thorough shampoo will remove dirt, sweat, grease, hairspray and other substances that coat the hair and scalp. The removal of such

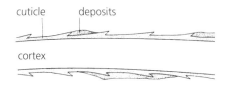

Dirt on the hair cuticle

substances is an essential part of the preparation for other hairdressing services, such as perming where any deposits of grease left on the hair shaft could block the perming chemicals and result in an unsuccessful perm. Shampooing is also used to remove the products used in other hairdressing services, including colouring and bleaching. At other times, the shampoo itself may include colouring ingredients that add colour to the hair. Whatever the purpose, a good shampoo will also be relaxing and enjoyable for the client.

Conditioning

Conditioning is used to restore the hair and scalp to a healthier state than previously. It is used to alleviate damage to the hair and scalp caused by both external factors, such as excessive use of heat when drying the hair, and internal factors, including poor diet and illness. Here are some of the factors that affect the condition of the hair and scalp and which can be improved by conditioning treatments:

External factors

- **Physical damage** – for example caused by harsh brushing or exposure to the sun and wind, etc.
- **Chemical damage** – for example caused by over-processing when perming hair, relaxing hair or bleaching hair, etc.

Internal factors

- **General health and lifestyle** – for example poor diet, the effects of medication, genetic conditions, pregnancy and stress.

How shampoos and conditioners work

Shampoos

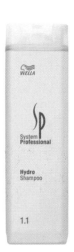

On its own water cannot dissolve the substances that become attached to the hair and scalp. Shampoo is added and rubbed into the head so that its cleaning ingredients and the dirt are agitated. The cleaners surround the particles of dirt, which are then rinsed away with water to leave the hair and scalp clean. Modern shampoos are very effective and only a little is required to clean the hair and scalp. A small amount, about 2–3 cm diameter, in the palm of your hand will usually be sufficient if thoroughly spread around the head and massaged effectively.

There are many different types of shampoo, but they can all be divided into four main groups:

- **Soap shampoos** – are not usually used in salons today, as the soap content leaves deposits of scum on the hair and scalp when they are used with hard water.

- **Soapless shampoos** – are used in most salons because they work well with both hard and soft water and do not leave deposits of scum.
- **Synthetic detergents** – the main ingredient in most soapless shampoos used today.
- **'2 in 1'** – products that act as a shampoo and as a frequent use conditioner.

Detergents

Water will not spread out thoroughly over the hair because weak electrical forces make the water molecules stick together to form water droplets. This electrical force is strongest at the surface of the water and is known as surface tension. Modern shampoos contain detergents that help to reduce the effect of these electrical forces, thereby reducing surface tension and allowing the water molecules to spread out and wet the hair. This means that you will also see detergents referred to as wetting agents.

A detergent molecule has two ends. One end is hydrophobic, meaning it repels water molecules (it attracts grease molecules instead), and the other end is hydrophilic, meaning it attracts water molecules. When the hair is shampooed, the hydrophobic ends of the detergent molecules are attracted to and surround each grease molecule (sebum). The grease molecules are then lifted away from the hair and scalp and suspended in the shampoo. This suspension is called an emulsion. Any dirt is held on the hair and scalp by the grease that is present, so when the grease lifts from the hair and scalp the dirt is removed too.

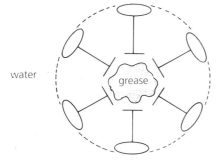

water   grease

Detergent molecules surrounding grease

A detergent molecule

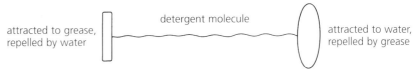

attracted to grease, repelled by water   detergent molecule   attracted to water, repelled by grease

'2 in 1' shampoos

'2 in 1' shampoos – so called because they act as a shampoo and as a frequent use conditioner – usually contain conditioner particles as well as detergent. The conditioner particles are a form of silicone, e.g. dimethicone, or positive electrically charged molecules. Hair has a slightly negative charge, which is greater where hair is damaged. Positive and negative electrical charges are attracted to each other, so when the hair is rinsed after shampooing the conditioning particles are released and attracted to the hair where they smooth the cuticle, especially where the hair is damaged. The conditioning particles are prevented from building up because shampooing removes the conditioning particles that were deposited previously.

Conditioners

As can be seen from the list of shampoo products above, most shampoos now contain some conditioning ingredients to provide for the conditioning required by most people. But other conditioners have been developed to meet clients' requirements when more specific or intensive conditioning is needed, such as after chemical processing.

Like 2 in 1 shampoos, most modern conditioners have positive electrically charged molecules that are attracted to the negatively charged hair. This provides what might be called an 'automatic' application of the conditioning molecules, as more are attracted to areas of damage where the negative charge in the hair is greater. These substances are called substantive conditioners. An additional benefit of applying positively charged conditioning molecules is that they cancel out the negative charge in the hair when they become attached and so reduce the static electricity that makes hair difficult to style and dress.

Other conditioners contain thickeners, restructurants and protein hydrolysates that combine with the polypeptide chains within the hair to create additional temporary linkages that help the hair regain strength and elasticity. Essentially conditioners re-balance the chemicals in the hair, support the structure and coat the cuticle to counteract the effects of physical and chemical damage.

The importance of water quality in shampooing and conditioning

Tip

Make your equipment last longer by keeping it free from lime scale deposits.

Hard water contains more calcium and/or magnesium salts than soft water. These substances react with sodium stearate in soap to form scum, or calcium magnesium stearate (soapless shampoos should be used in salons to avoid such problems). Whether an area has hard or soft water is a natural phenomenon of the geology of the local land. You might see mineral deposits form in kettles or around spray heads in salons in hard water areas. Distilled water should be used in steamers to avoid hard water deposits damaging the equipment.

The pH scale

The pH scale measures acidity and alkalinity ranging from pH1 to pH14. A pH of 1 indicates the strongest acid whilst a pH of 14 indicates the strongest alkaline; a pH of 7 is considered neutral. Understanding the pH scale is important in hairdressing because of the effects that some hairdressing chemicals have on the body's natural pH levels. The normal pH of the hair is pH 4.5–5.5 and the pH of the surface of the skin is pH 5–6, mildly acidic, caused by an oil produced in the skin called sebum. This acidic coating is called the skin's acid mantle. This mantle acts as a barrier to infection, slowing down the growth of bacteria and keeping the skin healthy. Raising the pH level above 5–6, which may happen if it is not re-balanced after certain hairdressing services that use alkaline products, e.g. perming, would reduce the effectiveness of this barrier and make infections more likely to occur. Some conditioning products are designed specifically to re-balance the natural pH of the hair and scalp after chemical services and are known as pH balanced conditioners.

APPROXIMATE pH VALUES OF VARIOUS SUBSTANCES

Acid	0.1–6.9
Alkali	7.1–14.0
Neutral solution	7.0
Normal hair/scalp	4.5–5.5
Pre-perm shampoo	7.0
pH-balanced shampoo/ conditioner	4.5–5.5

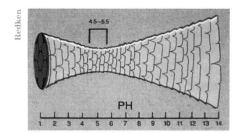

How pH affects the hair

Hair is also affected by the level of acidity and alkalinity. When it is slightly alkaline the cuticles lift and the hair shaft wells, however if it is mildly acidic the cuticles close up. Very strong readings towards either acid or alkaline will cause the hair to break down. The pH of a substance can be measured using pH papers, or Litmus papers that change colour to indicate pH value.

The pH scale

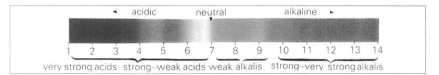

Selecting the correct product

Shampooing and conditioning is very similar for men and women. The same process is used and the same products are usually equally suitable, but some differences do occur. Men tend to want products that contain less perfume and the packaging of retail products for men is designed specifically to attract them. However, the choice of product is really made on the basis of more scientific factors, such as the needs of the hair and scalp.

Selecting shampoo products

The choice of the correct shampoo depends on several factors.

- **Water quality** – as we have seen earlier the minerals in hard water will react with sodium stearate in soap to form scum. Soapless shampoos that do not produce scum should therefore be used in salons.
- **Services planned** – the services that will follow the shampooing process must be considered to make sure that the shampoo used is compatible with the forthcoming service, e.g. pre-perm shampoos should be used before a perm.
- **The reason for the shampoo** – why is the shampoo being performed? Is it to clean, remove colour products, add colour products or condition?
- **The frequency of the shampoo** – hair that is washed more often is usually less dirty and greasy, so milder shampoos designed for frequent use should be used.
- **The hair type and texture** – coarse and thick hair needs a shampoo that will make it more pliable, while fine hair benefits from a shampoo that adds body.
- **Hair condition** – a list of common hair conditions and examples of their treatment is provided in Chapter 2, 'Client care for men'. Here are some popular shampoos, their ingredients and uses:

– *Medicated* – to maintain healthy hair and scalp.

– *Treatment* – many different shampoos are developed to treat different problems, like over-greasy hair and scalp or dandruff. Ingredients include selenium sulphide or zinc for dandruff.

– *Pre-perm* – used before a perm to remove substances that could affect the perming process.

– *'2 in 1'* – acts as a shampoo and as a frequent use conditioner. Contains conditioner particles that are positively electrically charged to be attracted to the hair, especially where the hair is damaged.

– *Egg* – egg white is used to improve over-greasy conditions and egg yolk is used for dry hair.

– *Camomile* – used to brighten blond hair. Can be effective against greasy conditions.

– *Coconut* – used for dry hair. Helps to smooth the hair and improve its elasticity.

– *Lemon* – used for over-greasy hair. The citrus ingredients cut through the grease and the slightly acidic pH closes the hair cuticle and makes the hair shine.

Selecting conditioning products

There are two main types on conditioner:

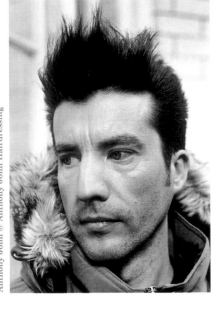

Anthony John @ Anthony John Hairdressing

- **Surface conditioners** – these add gloss and shine to the hair by smoothing the cuticle, which also makes the hair more manageable. They remain on the surface of the hair and do not enter the cortex. They include reconditioning creams and oils and dressing creams and lotions and contain ingredients such as vegetable and mineral oils, lanolin, lecithin and acetic acid.

- **Penetrating conditioners** – these enter the cortex through capillary action, i.e. the conditioner is drawn into the hair shaft through the tiny spaces in the hair structure. These conditioners can repair the cortical fibres, introduce moisture and smooth the cuticle. They contain ingredients such as protein hydrolysates, humectants (substances that hold water) and moisturisers.

The choice of correct conditioner also depends on several factors:

- **Services planned and carried out** – the services that will follow the conditioning process must be considered to make sure that the conditioner used is compatible with the forthcoming service, e.g. only use conditioners designed for use before perming or the chemicals in the perm will not be able to enter the hair shaft. Some conditioners are used after other hairdressing services to stop the chemical process – anti-oxidants – and re-balance pH levels – pH balancers.

- **The reason for the conditioner** – why is it being performed? Is it to protect the hair before chemical services, add moisture or help reconstruct the cortical fibres?

- **The frequency of the conditioner** – hair that is washed and conditioned more often is usually less dry, so conditioners for frequent use should be used.

- **The hair type and texture** – coarse and thick hair needs a conditioner that will make it more pliable. Fine hair is improved by conditioners that contain catatonic polymers that add body.

- **Hair condition** – a list of common hair conditions and examples of their treatment is provided in Chapter 2, 'Client care for men'. Here are some popular conditioners, their ingredients and uses:

  - *Anti-oxidants* – conditioners used after chemical processing to stop oxidation and neutralise alkaline

  - *pH balancers* – used after chemical processing to restore pH levels

  - *Pre-perm conditioners* – used before a perm to even out porosity and improve the perming process

  - *'2 in 1'* – acts as a shampoo and as a frequent use conditioner. Contains conditioner particles that are positively electrically charged that are attracted to the hair, especially where the hair is damaged. Easy and quick for clients to use at home.

  - *Lacquer* – help resist the ingress of moisture and to shape the hair. Can smooth the cuticle and enhance the glossy appearance.

  - *Restructurants* – these penetrate the hair shaft and help repair and support damaged cortical fibres, making the hair more pliable and able to be styled.

  - *Other dressings* – help add and retain moisture and smooth the cuticles.

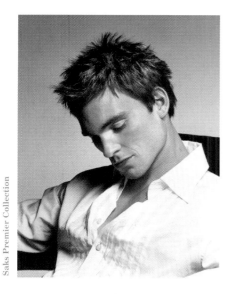

Saks Premier Collection

Consultation prior to shampooing and conditioning

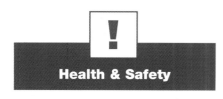

Health & Safety

You must carry out a thorough consultation to ensure that you identify any adverse conditions of the hair or skin that may be present. It is particularly important to establish whether a suspected infection or infestation is present, as this would prevent you from shampooing or conditioning the hair. (This area is covered more fully in Chapter 2, 'Client care for men').

It is important to consider the client's hair type, texture and condition and the other hairdressing services required when choosing the product, water temperature and shampoo massage techniques to be used. You must give careful consideration to each of the following factors before you start work:

- Why does the client want the shampoo or conditioning treatment?

- Look for signs of broken skin, abnormalities on the skin, or any unusual facial features or beard growth patterns.

- Is the hair fine, medium or coarse?

- Is the hair growth dense or sparse – does the density of growth vary around the head?

- Determine which other hairdressing services are to be provided following the shampooing or conditioning.

Preparation for shampooing and conditioning

- Carry out your consultation with the client. Look for signs of broken skin, and any abnormalities on the skin.
- Determine the client's wishes and confirm what is to be done.
- Gather together all the products, towels, tools and equipment you will require before you begin work.
- The client should be gowned correctly for the type of basin you are using. A back wash basin requires a gown and then a clean towel placed across the client's back, a front wash basin requires a gown and a towel across the client's chest with a second towel across his back and over the first towel. Make sure the towels are tucked in at the neck to prevent them from falling when the client leans forward.
- Position the client in the chair correctly so that his head can be positioned comfortably over the basin. Ensure his head is correctly supported by the back wash basin when using this method.
- Carefully comb the hair through before commencing. Look out for areas of sparse growth, scarring or other unusual features you may not have seen earlier.

Shampooing and conditioning techniques

The following manual massage techniques are commonly used when shampooing hair.

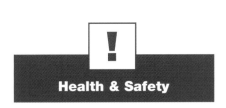

Health & Safety

Make sure that your fingernails are not too long before performing manual scalp massage, as long fingernails could dig in to the skin.

- **Effleurage** is a circular, stroking movement where the fingers move freely around the head. It is the foundation of all good massage and is used to induce relaxation, particularly at the start and the completion of the shampooing procedure.
- **Rotary** movements are similar to effleurage movements because the fingers make small circular, or rotary movements on the head. It also has similarities with petrissage, however, as the fingers move less across the scalp during each movement than they do in effleurage. Rotary is good for cleaning the scalp and it creates an invigorating sensation for the client.
- **Petrissage** is performed through a mixture of pinching, kneading and rolling movements across the scalp. It is applied with both hands, which often work together to gently lift the skin between the fingers and thumbs, where it is squeezed, rolled and pinched with a gentle but firm pressure.
- **Friction**, or vibration, is a rubbing movement often used with friction hair tonics in scalp massage. It has a stimulating affect on the scalp and produces an invigorating sensation for the client.

The effleurage, petrissage and friction massage techniques are also commonly used when providing scalp massage as part of conditioning services. This form of scalp massage is explained fully in Chapter 9, 'Scalp massage'.

A shampooing and conditioning procedure

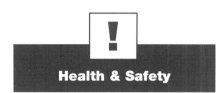
1 Ensure that your client is correctly gowned and protected.
2 Prepare the hair, as required.
3 Check that the client is comfortable.
4 Turn on the cold water first and then the hot water until the correct temperature is achieved. Test the temperature on the back of your hand.
5 Check that the flow of water is not too strong or water will splash off the client's head and wet their clothes and the salon.
6 Maintain your hand in the flow of water during rinsing to check that the water temperature remains stable.
7 Thoroughly wet the hair, controlling the flow to keep the client's clothes, and your own clothes and the rest of the salon dry. Turn off the water.

Wetting the hair

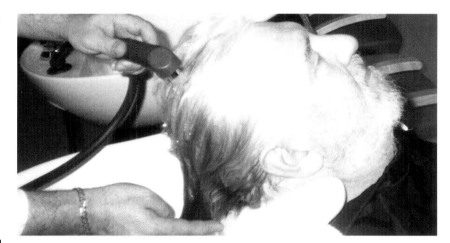

8 Apply sufficient shampoo for the length and density of hair into the palm of your hand (a 2–3 cm diameter amount is usually sufficient). Spread the shampoo over the palms of both hands and then distribute it throughout the hair and scalp using effleurage.
9 Use light effleurage movements to relax the client, each hand moving in alternate directions (imagine you are drawing a zigzag pattern across the head). Work slowly and carefully to let the client become accustomed to the sensation.
10 Move the fingers back towards the temples then make small circular rotary movements working back across the head to the crown area. Repeat this series of movements several times working up to the top of the head.
11 Slide your fingers down the back of the head and make spiralling rotary movements with each hand down to the nape, moving back up towards the crown after each stroke.
12 Place the fingers on the front hairline. Using light pinching and squeezing petrissage movements, work back along the head to the crown. Slide the fingers back down to the temples and then work back up towards the top of the crown, using the pinching movements as before. Make sure you cover all of the head.
13 Slide back down to the nape area. Using the middle fingers of each hand make two deep, rotating petrissage movements then

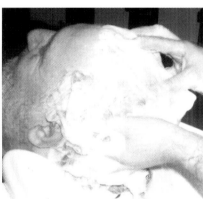

Effleurage

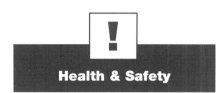

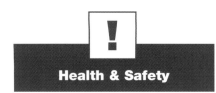

Health & Safety

Always make sure you remove shampoo and other hairdressing products from your hands and dry them carefully. Gently pat your hands when drying them. Failure to follow these steps can make your hands dry and sore and can lead to dermatitis.

continue this movement up across the head and to the temples. Repeat this movement several times.

14 Slide your fingers back to the front hairline. Using your fingertips apply a light friction movement and work back across the head to the crown and down the back to the nape. Repeat these movements from the sides to the nape. You should develop a gentle rhythm to make the movement enjoyable for the client.

15 Complete the massage routine with gentle sweeping effleurage movements across the head.

16 Repeat steps 4 and 5 and rinse the hair thoroughly.

17 Apply more shampoo and repeat steps 8–16 if required.

18 A surface conditioner can now be applied, if required.

19 After the final rinsing, turn off the water and replace the spray head. Wrap the hair in a towel and gently remove any surplus water. Reposition the client, check that dirt, grease and any products have been removed from the hair and scalp and that all shampoo has been rinsed out.

20 Comb the client's hair back away from his face using a wide toothed comb to avoid pulling the hair.

Health and safety

Everyone in the salon has a duty to work safely and keep his or her environment safe. It is important to consider health and safety when shampooing and conditioning because of the risks associated with using hot water and electricity. Here are some important health and safety factors that you must consider when providing shampooing and conditioning services:

- If the client has any cuts or abrasions on his face, or you suspect that an infection or infestation is present, the work must not be carried out.

- Always make sure you remove shampoo and other hairdressing products from your hands and dry them carefully. Gently pat your hands when drying them. Failure to follow these steps can make your hands dry and sore and can lead to dermatitis.

- Always turn on the cold water first and add the hot water afterwards. Check the temperature of the water on you own hand and keep checking it to prevent scalding.

- Electrical equipment must always be handled and used with care in accordance with the manufacturer's instructions.

- *Never* use or place electrical equipment near water.

- *Do not* go near electrical equipment that is lying in water – isolate the mains power first.

- Visually check that electrical equipment is safe to use before commencing work – check that the cable has not frayed or been pulled and that the plug is not loose.

- Pay attention to the position of cables when using and storing electrical equipment.

- Only use clean tools and equipment.
- Make sure that you know the whereabouts of your salon's first-aid kit. Keep yourself up to date with your salon's first-aid and accident procedures.
- Electrical equipment must be regularly tested and given a certificate of testing to confirm that it is safe for use. Your salon owner will ensure that this is carried out, as required.
- Maintain spray heads and steamers correctly and keep them free from lime scale.
- Make sure you know where the mains water stopcock and mains electricity switch are so that you can turn of the supplies quickly if problems occur.

Activities

1   Find out whether the water in your salon is temporarily or permanently soft or hard.
2   Find out where the water stop cock and main electricity switch are located in your salon. Make sure you know how to turn them off in case of an emergency, such as a burst pipe or electrical fire.
3   Examine your colleagues' hair and let them examine yours to assess each others' hair and scalp condition. Write down your findings and check your results with your manager or tutor.

Check your knowledge

1   Describe dry shampooing.
2   What are the main differences in shampooing in barber's shops when compared with unisex or women's salons?
3   What is the main purpose of shampooing?
4   List two causes of physical damage to the hair.
5   List the four main types of shampoo.
6   Describe how a detergent works.
7   What is the meaning of the term 'hydrophobic'?
8   What is one benefit of using a substantive conditioner?
9   Provide two reasons for the importance of considering the hardness of water in shampooing and conditioning.
10   What is the normal pH value of skin?
11   What is the correct type of shampoo to use on greasy hair?
12   Describe the type of hair that benefits most from a conditioner containing catatonic polymers.
13   What should you look out for on the client's skin during consultation?
14   Describe the rotary massage movement.
15   What is one effect of the friction massage movement?
16   Why should the cold water be turned on first?
17   Why is it important to keep the shower spray heads clear, especially in hard water areas?

Cutting facial hair using basic techniques

4

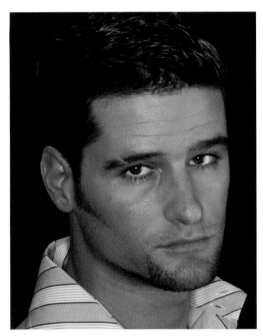

Forfex Professional

Learning objectives

The beard and moustache have played an important role in men's fashions throughout the ages. At one time most men wore a beard, a moustache or long sideburns, but the popularity of the clean-shaven appearance increased following the introduction of safety razors and electric shavers. Today there is again a marked increase in the popularity of beards and moustaches, especially with young men, who now often wear short styles such as a goatee beard.

This chapter looks at the basic techniques used for cutting facial hair to maintain existing shapes and covers the following topics:

- **cutting and styling facial hair – including traditional and current shapes**
- **consultation prior to cutting facial hair**
- **tools and equipment**
- **preparation for cutting facial hair**
- **cutting techniques**
- **a facial haircutting procedure**
- **finishing**
- **health and safety**

Cutting and styling facial hair

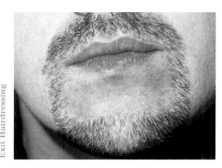

Exit Hairdressing

The purpose of cutting facial hair is both to shorten the hair and to style it into shape. This is achieved with scissors or clippers, which are usually used with a comb to perform cutting techniques described as 'scissors-over-comb' or 'clippers-over-comb'.

Sometimes clippers are used with a comb attachment such that the hair is cut at a predetermined length. This attachment is relatively easy to use, and has become popular with many men for keeping their beards and moustaches in shape between salon visits.

Traditional and current beard and moustache shapes

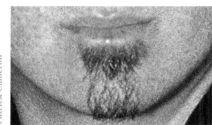

Patrick Cameron

Over the years many beard, moustache and sideburn shapes have been developed. Some can be described as traditional, as men first started wearing them many hundreds of years ago. Some of these traditional shapes may also be described as being current shapes, because men today are still wearing the shape or because the shape is currently fashionable. Yet other shapes are new, as they have only just been developed for the look that men like today: these too can be described as current shapes.

The barber must be familiar with many different traditional and current shapes, and able to visualise the right shape for each client and advise him accordingly. Here are some beard and moustache shapes for you to consider.

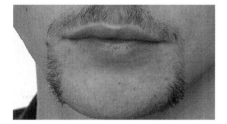

Charlie Miller

In the past beards, moustaches and sideburns would often be dressed into different styles using various dressings, pomades or wax. These made the hair very stiff and enabled the wearer to create intricate styles, such as the traditional handlebar moustache. Dressing creams, pomades, waxes and gels are sometimes used to style facial hair today, but usually only to smooth stray hairs or to create definition or texture on longer beards.

Consultation prior to cutting facial hair

When maintaining the beard, moustache or sideburn shape it is important to consider the client's face shape and hairstyle. You should think of these as being integrated parts of one style, or one total look and trim the beard or moustache shape to suit.

Men are often very particular about their beard, so before you start work carefully consider each of the following factors.

- What does the client want?
- Why does he have a beard or moustache?
- Look for signs of broken skin, abnormalities on the skin, or any unusual facial features or beard growth patterns.

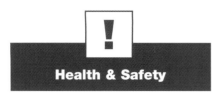

Before you start cutting, you must carry out a thorough consultation. Be sure to identify any adverse conditions of the hair or skin that may be present. It is particularly important to establish whether you have reason to suspect any infection or infestation, as this would prevent you from cutting the facial hair. (This area is covered more fully in Chapter 2.)

Tip

It is usually far better to go *with* the direction of beard growth than to go against it, especially when cutting strong growth patterns.

Tip

Especially with new clients, it is particularly important when cutting existing beard shapes to look for variations in the density of growth: the hair may have been left long in some areas to disguise very sparse growth or to cover a scar. Cutting the hair too short in these areas would expose the skin, and might well annoy or embarrass the client.

- Is the beard hair fine, medium or coarse?
- Is the beard growth dense or sparse? Does the density of beard growth vary around the face?
- Pay attention to the client's face shape.
- Pay attention to the length and shape of his hairstyle.

Hair growth patterns

Hair growth patterns are the way in which individual hairs or a section of the beard may grow in a particular direction. Hair growth patterns must be identified because they determine both the shape that can be created and the techniques that you should use. Some clients have very strong hair growth patterns in their beard, such as hair whorls: these should be cut by following the direction of hair growth around the whorl.

Texture

The texture of hair in a beard can be fine, medium or coarse. Young men usually have fine facial hair, but as men get older their facial hair often becomes much coarser. Fine hair is usually easier to cut, but some fuller styles will be more difficult to create. Coarse hair is often more difficult to cut, and is liable to fly in all directions during cutting – extra care must be taken to protect the client's and your own eyes. Coarser hair lends itself to many different beard shapes, but you must also consider the density of growth.

Density

Hair density is the amount of hair that grows in a given area of skin. Some men have a very dense beard growth, which is sometimes known as a blue beard because the density of growth gives the skin a blue tinge which remains even after shaving. Indeed, this could be the main reason why the client has grown a beard.

The density of beard growth often varies around the face. Some men have dense growth around their chin, cheeks and top lip, but sparse growth between the bottom lip and chin. Others have dense growth only on their top lip. Yet others have dense growth everywhere except on the top lip. And in others the density of growth may be very sparse, preventing the client from growing certain beard or moustache shapes.

Face shape and facial features

It is important to identify the client's face shape and consider his facial features so that you can avoid damage to the skin and so that you can maintain the most suitable shape. You must make careful note of the following:

- the size and position of the mouth
- the width of the top lip

Health & Safety

Take extra care when cutting very coarse or dense beards. The hair is liable to fly in all directions while it is being cut. Make sure the client's eyes are well protected with clean cottonwool pads or tissues, and keep your own face well away from the work. If you find the hair is very strong and springy, you may need to wear safety glasses to protect your eyes.

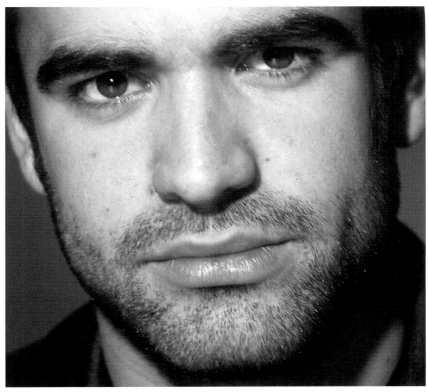

EXIT Hairdressing

- the shape of the nose
- the shape of the jaw and chin
- any unusual features, such as moles, dimples or scarring

Different face shapes require different beard and moustache shapes. These are explained in more detail in Chapter 13, 'Designing facial hair shapes'.

Tools and equipment

Tips

- Use the mirror regularly during cutting to ensure that the shape is centralised and symmetrical.
- Pay particular attention to where the beard or sideburns meet the hairstyle, and ensure that they blend together.

Read the section on haircutting tools in Chapter 5, 'Cutting men's hair' (page 79): these rules also apply to tools for cutting facial hair.

Tools

All haircutting tools must be well-balanced, sharp, clean, and safe to use. Here are the main tools required for cutting facial hair.

Scissors

Scissors are available in different sizes, ranging from 10cm to 18cm in length. Most barbers prefer scissors around 15cm, but you need to find out what feels comfortable given the size of your hand and the job you are doing.

Thinning scissors are used to remove bulk without removing length.

Clippers

Clippers may be either hand-operated or electric. Hand clippers are not usually used today unless electricity is unavailable, such as during a power cut.

Electric clippers may be powered by either mains electricity or rechargeable batteries. They are the preferred choice today because of their power, accuracy and convenience when compared to hand clippers. They are used to create outlines or when using clippers-over-comb techniques. Detachable comb attachments are also available, which give a wide range of predetermined cutting lengths. These allow for very fast removal of hair and are sometimes used to reduce the length of the beard, which is then finished with scissors and clippers (without the comb attached).

Razors

Razors are sometimes used to shave part of the face, to emphasise the beard or moustache style. Disposable-blade razors are best because they are more hygienic.

Equipment

The client should be seated in an adjustable chair which can be positioned so that the client can recline comfortably. The chair should have a headrest and the height of the chair should be adjustable so that you do not have to bend uncomfortably.

Preparation for cutting facial hair

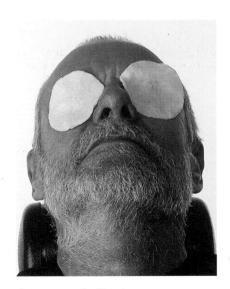

A prepared client

1   Carry out your consultation with the client. Look for signs of broken skin, abnormalities on the skin, and unusual beard growth patterns.

2   Determine the client's wishes and confirm what is to be done.

3   Position the client in a reclining chair so that you can work on the beard. Ensure you provide support for his head.

4   Before you begin work, gather together all the tools and equipment you will need.

5   Gown the client and place a clean towel across his chest, tucked in at the neck.

6   Protect the client's eyes with tissue or cottonwool pads that have been moistened with warm water. The moisture helps the pads stay in place and will be soothing for the eyes. Make sure the tissue or pads are not *too* wet, however: they should be nearly dry.

7   Carefully comb the beard, disentangling the hair as necessary. Look out for areas of sparse growth, scarring or other unusual features you may not have seen earlier.

Cutting techniques

The following cutting techniques are commonly used when cutting facial hair to shape.

Scissors-over-comb

Scissors-over-comb cutting is performed by first lifting a section of hair, and then cutting straight across. When cutting beards and moustaches you should take small sections of hair: these are usually lifted with the comb as the hair is quite short. Some barbers, especially when working on longer hair, use the tips of their scissors to lift the sections of hair: the hair is then picked up on the comb and positioned ready for cutting.

Scissors-over-comb is often used to create graduated effects by adjusting the angle and length of each section. Be sure to use the fine teeth of the comb and the tips of the scissors when working around the lips.

Scissors-over-comb technique

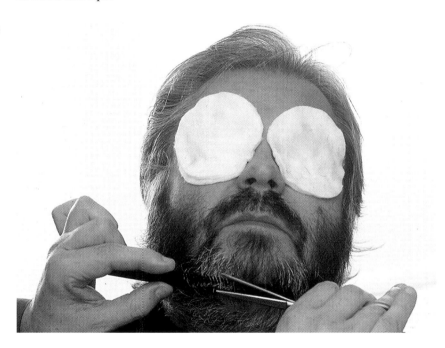

Clippers-over-comb

Clippers-over-comb cutting is often used instead of scissors-over-comb techniques, especially on longer, coarser and denser beards. Generally, the same effects possible with scissors can be achieved using clippers. Smaller clippers are easier to use on moustaches and when working around the lips, as the blades are smaller and more accurate.

Freehand cutting

Freehand cutting is the cutting of hair without first taking the hair into a section or holding the hair in place with the comb or hand. It is often used to remove individual hairs or small amounts of hair when finishing a style, and is usually performed with the tips of the scissors. When cutting beards and moustaches it is used to smooth the outline shape and remove stray hairs.

Razoring

Razoring is sometimes used to create clean outlines and emphasise a shape. It is performed with a razor, which may be either an open razor or a safety razor. Disposable-blade razors are best because they are more hygienic. Electric razors are also sometimes used.

Cutting procedures

The long beard

1 Protect the client's clothes and eyes.
2 Comb the beard carefully, disentangling the hair where required.
3 Start at one side of your client (it does not matter which), and begin cutting the beard hair using the scissors- or clippers-over-comb technique (b). Start in the area where the sideburns join the head hair. Make sure you blend the beard and head hair to suit the overall look.
4 Keep working down the side of the face (c), cutting the hair to the length determined by the beard shape. Do not cut the moustache at this stage. If the beard is to be longer towards the chin you should gradually increase the length as you work down the beard.
5 Repeat this on the other side. As the shape develops, keep looking in the mirror to make sure that the beard is symmetrical.
6 Move to the centre of the beard and cut the hair using scissors- or clippers-over-comb techniques, as before (d). Take small sections, blending the two sides into the final shape. If you wish to create a pointed beard, angle your comb towards the point of the chin; otherwise blend the two sides together to create an even, continuous effect.

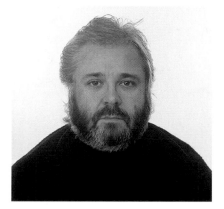

(a) Before cutting

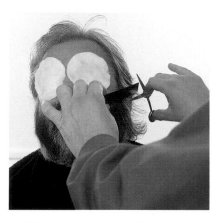

(b) Starting at one side

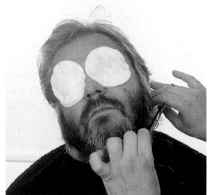

(c) Cutting down the side

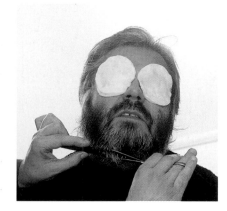

(d) Cutting in the centre

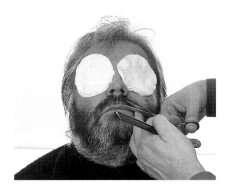

(e) Outlining the moustache

7 Move to one side of the moustache. Carefully outline the moustache along the top lip to create the required shape, using the tips of your scissors or the clippers (e). Use the fingers of your other hand to guide and support the scissors or clippers whilst cutting.

8 Repeat this on the other side of the moustache (f).

9 Using your comb, lift small sections of the moustache hair and cut this to the required length. Use the tips of your scissors and small, careful movements (g).

10 Blend the moustache into the beard, as required by the overall shape.

11 Lift the client's chin and carefully cut the neck outline to the correct height (h). This outline may be graduated to create a natural effect, or cut into a clean line for a more defined look. The centre of the outline (below the chin) should be cut slightly higher than at the sides to compensate for the skin in the centre moving further up as the head goes back. The difference should be about 1cm. This will appear level when the head is returned to its normal position.

12 Cut the other outlines on the cheeks, chin or above the moustache, as required. Refer to the mirror to keep the outlines symmetrical.

13 Shave the areas outside the outlines if necessary (see Chapter 11).

14 Graduate the outlines to blend them with the skin, where required (i).

15 Finish the shape by combing the hair into place (j).

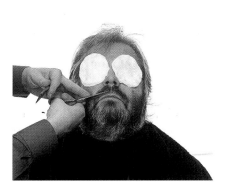

(f) Outlining the other side

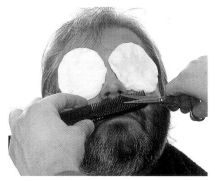

(g) Cutting the moustache

Tip

Cut the centre of the outline below the chin slightly higher than at the sides to compensate for the skin moving up whilst the head is held back.

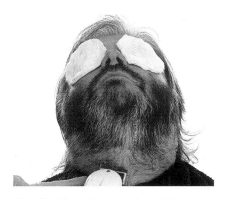

(h) Cutting the neck outline

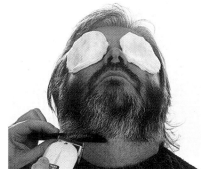

(i) Graduating outlines

(j) The finished look

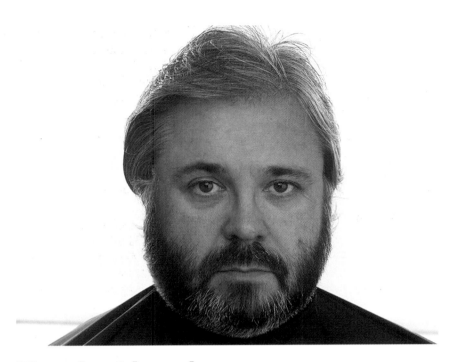

The short beard

1 Protect the client's clothes and eyes, as before (a).
2 Comb the beard carefully, disentangling the hair where required.
3 Start at one side of your client and begin cutting the beard hair, using the scissors- or clippers-over-comb technique or using a clipper attachment. Again, make sure you blend the beard and head hair to suit the overall look.
4 Keep working down the side of the face, cutting the hair to the length determined by the beard shape. Do not cut the moustache at this stage. As with the long beard, if the beard shape is to be longer towards the chin you should gradually increase the length as you work down the beard.
5 Repeat this on the other side. Keep looking in the mirror to make sure that the beard is symmetrical.
6 Move to the centre of the beard and cut the hair, using scissors- or clippers-over-comb techniques or the clipper attachment (b). Blend the two sides into the final shape. If you wish to create a pointed beard, angle your comb towards the point of the chin; otherwise blend the two sides together to create an even, continuous effect (c).

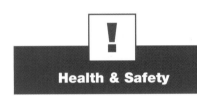

Health & Safety

● Always protect the client's eyes from hairs, which may fly up during cutting, especially on very coarse beards. Keep your own face away from your work; wear safety glasses for protection.

● To ensure the client's comfort, remove excess hair cuttings from his face and neck at frequent intervals.

Tip

The procedure for cutting a short beard into shape is basically the same as for cutting a long beard, but many barbers use a clipper attachment to first cut the beard to a predetermined length, and then finish with scissors and comb.

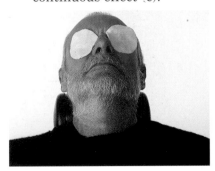

(a) Before cutting

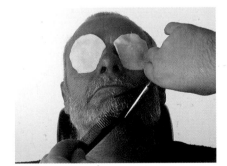

(b) Cutting the centre of the beard

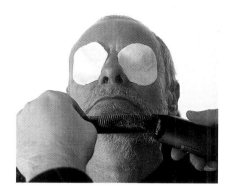

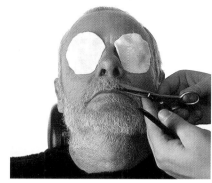

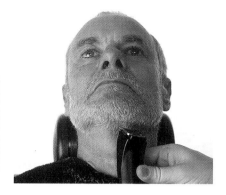

(c) Using clippers-over-comb for the centre of the beard

(d) Cutting the moustache

(e) Cutting the neck outline

Tips

- When determining the correct height for the neck outline you should consider the overall shape and length of the beard. If the outline is too low it will be visible below the chin when viewed from the front: this can appear untidy. If it is too high, however, the outline will be visible across the side of the face. The best height is usually about 2cm below the jawline, but always consider your client's wishes.

- Outlines can be achieved by cutting the hair either with close-cutting clippers or with an electric razor. The outline hair may also be removed completely by shaving with a razor, which should be used following the shaving procedure described in Chapter 11.

7 Move to one side of the moustache. Carefully outline the moustache along the top lip to create the required shape, using the tips of your scissors or the clippers (d).

8 Repeat this on the other side of the moustache.

9 Using your comb, lift small sections of the moustache hair and cut this to the required length. The clipper attachment is not really suitable here.

10 Blend the moustache into the beard, as required by the overall shape.

11 Lift the client's chin and carefully cut the neck outline to the correct height (e).

12 Cut the other outlines on the cheeks, chin or above the moustache, as required. Refer to the mirror to keep the outlines symmetrical.

13 If necessary, shave the areas outside the outlines (see Chapter 11).

14 Graduate the outlines to blend them with the skin, where required.

15 Finish the shape by combing the hair into place (f).

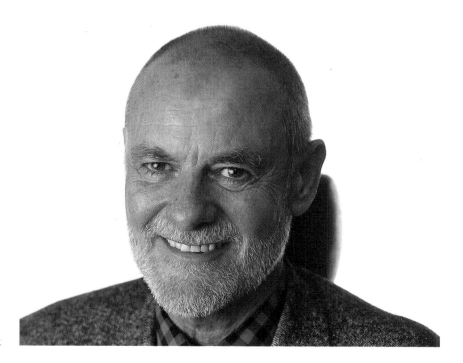

(f) The finished look

Finishing

After cutting a styling aid may be applied to help smooth the hair, particularly on longer beard and moustache shapes. Use the mirror regularly to check the balance and symmetry of the shape as you dress it.

Comb the client's head hair into style, if required, and allow the client to see your work. Provide advice on after-care, as required.

Health and safety

Everyone in the salon has a duty to work safely and keep the salon environment safe. When cutting facial hair it is important to consider health and safety because of the risks associated with using electricity and the risk of cutting the skin.

Here are some important health and safety factors that you must consider when providing haircutting services:

Avoid infection

- If the client has any cuts or abrasions on his face, or you suspect that an infection or infestation is present, you must not carry out the work.
- Pay special attention to hygiene when cutting facial hair, because of the risk of cross-infection through open cuts.
- Use only clean tools and equipment.

Protect the eyes

- Always protect the client's eyes from hairs using tissues or cottonwool pads. Keep your own face away from your work; if necessary, wear safety glasses.

Work safely with razors

- Open and safety razors have very sharp blades and must always be handled and used with great care.
- When it is not being used or when it is being carried, always close the handle to protect the blade of an open razor.
- Never place razors or other cutting tools in your pockets.
- Always sterilise a fixed-blade razor before each use.
- When using a detachable-blade open razor, always use a new blade for each new client.
- Used razor blades, called sharps, must be disposed of correctly in accordance with your salon policy. Soiled disposable materials should be placed in sealed plastic bags for removal.

Work safely with electricity

- Always handle and use electrical equipment with care, and in accordance with the manufacturers' instructions.

- Never place or use electric clippers or other electrical equipment near water.
- Do not go near electrical equipment that is lying in water – first switch off the power at the mains.
- Before commencing work, visually check that electrical equipment is safe to use. Check that the cable has not frayed or been pulled, and that the plug is not loose.
- When using and storing electrical equipment, pay attention to the position of cables.
- Never overload sockets. Do not plug too many items of electrical equipment into the same socket.
- Follow the manufacturer's instructions for the care of your clippers. To avoid damage, be sure to clean and lubricate the blades regularly.
- Electrical equipment must be regularly tested, and given a certificate of testing confirming that it is safe for use. The salon owner will ensure that this is carried out, as required.

Be prepared for accidents

- Make sure that you know the whereabouts of your salon's first-aid kit.
- Keep yourself up to date with your salon's first-aid and accident procedures.

Activity

Visit a library or use the Internet to research the different types of traditional beard shapes that have been popular in different eras over the past 2000 years. Compare these to shapes worn today and note the key differences.

Check your knowledge

1 Describe the differences between traditional and current beard and moustache shapes.
2 Describe a hair whorl.
3 Describe how hair density affects the choice of facial hair shape.
4 List five facial features that must be considered before cutting facial hair.
5 Describe the beard and moustache shapes most suited to a client with a long face.
6 State when razors would be used in cutting beards and moustaches.
7 List two reasons for using freehand techniques when cutting beards and moustaches into shape.
8 Describe the special safety precautions that must be taken when cutting facial hair that are not normally required when cutting hair.
9 Describe how to check that electrical equipment is safe before use.
10 Where should razors never be placed?

Cutting men's hair using basic techniques

5

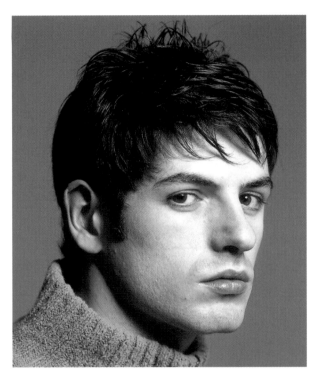

Learning objectives

Competent haircutting is the foundation of all good hairdressing, and cutting skills are amongst the most important that any hairdresser has. These skills are particularly important to the barber because most clients visiting the barber's shop want their hair cut. Indeed, some barbers perform few, if any, other services.

This chapter looks at the basic techniques the barber uses for cutting men's hair. It covers the following topics:

- **cutting and styling men's hair – including outlines, sideburns and neckline shapes**
- **consultation prior to cutting men's hair**
- **tools and equipment**
- **preparation for cutting men's hair**
- **cutting techniques – including wet and dry cutting**
- **cutting procedures**
- **finishing**
- **health and safety**

Cutting and styling men's hair

The main purpose of cutting hair is to style the hair into shape. Both the hair length and the hair thickness can be removed, either to create a completely new look or just to trim the client's current look back into shape. Cutting also removes any split ends (fragilitas crinium) that may be present, thereby improving the condition and appearance of the hair.

Men's haircutting is achieved with scissors and clippers, although razors are also sometimes used as required to shave the outlines, thin the hair or produce textured effects. Club cutting with scissors-over-comb and clippers-over-comb techniques is most often required.

Sometimes the clippers are used with a comb attachment that positions the blades to cut the hair at a predetermined length. These are particularly useful for creating short looks on longer hair, as the long hair can be removed quickly and easily to produce a rough shape ready for finishing.

The haircut

The haircut has an important role in hairdressing because it is the basis on which all other hairstyling takes place. It determines how the hair can be later dressed and styled, and how easy that styling will be. A good haircut design should make the client look and feel good and will be easy for him to manage. Indeed, most men want a style that is 'easy to maintain'.

There are many similarities between cutting men's hair and women's hair. Often the same cutting techniques can be used and sometimes men and women wear the same looks, but there are

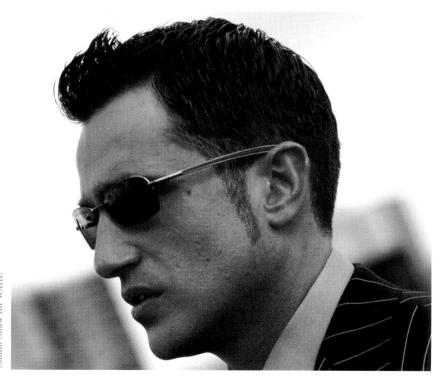

Simon Shaw for WAHL

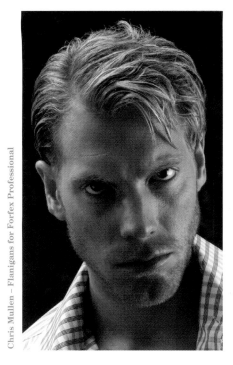

Chris Mullen – Flanigans for Forfex Professional

usually subtle differences in the shapes that are required and in the methods that are used to achieve them. Facial hair, dense hair growth on the neck and male-pattern alopecia (baldness), which usually occur in men only, must be especially considered.

There are also distinct differences between masculine and feminine shapes. Masculine shapes are usually more square and angular and are suited to most men, while feminine shapes tend to be fuller and more rounded. Taller, less full, or leaner shapes are also more flattering on most men, so minimal thickness at the back and sides is often required. Remember that these are just basic principles, however: they should be adapted to take account of factors such as the client's wishes, his face shape and his hair growth patterns. The client consultation will help you determine which of these shapes is best suited to the particular client.

Most men, and many women too, wear short layered looks. These are popular because they require minimal blow-styling and dressing, and so are easy for clients to maintain. Many of these haircuts are so short that the styling details are quite subtle: precise cutting movements and accurate cutting angles are required. Often only very small amounts of hair are removed at a time until the desired effect is achieved – great care is needed, as the hair is too short to hide any mistakes. Most short layered looks are graduated at the back and sides. The outlines of these haircuts are often emphasised, and these require careful attention.

Cutting outlines

Outlining with scissors

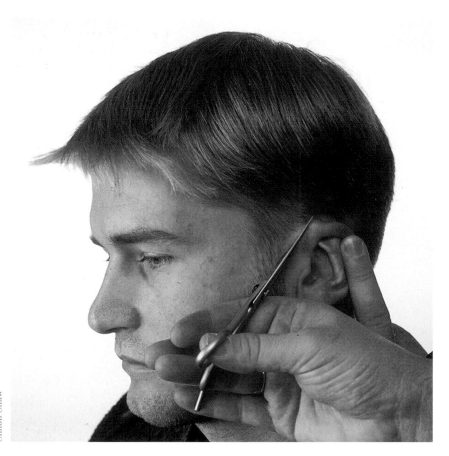

Simon Shaw

Many men have dense hair growth outside the natural hairline, particularly on the face and in the nape areas, whereas most women have soft, natural hairlines with few hairs growing outside. On women the outline usually requires little further definition, but on most men the haircut must be outlined or it appears untidy and unfinished.

In the past, outlines were cut with scissors and by shaving. The shaving was performed with an open razor and was used to remove all unwanted hair from outside the haircut outline. This produced a smooth, close finish that helped to extend the life of the haircut as the hair took longer to grow back. Today, outlines are usually shaped with the points of the scissors and with electric clippers, which can cut the hair nearly as close as when shaved. Shaving is still used sometimes, when a particularly close finish is required. Many barbers use both scissors and clippers throughout the outlining of a haircut. The choice of tool and technique is determined both by the needs of the haircut and by the barber's personal preference.

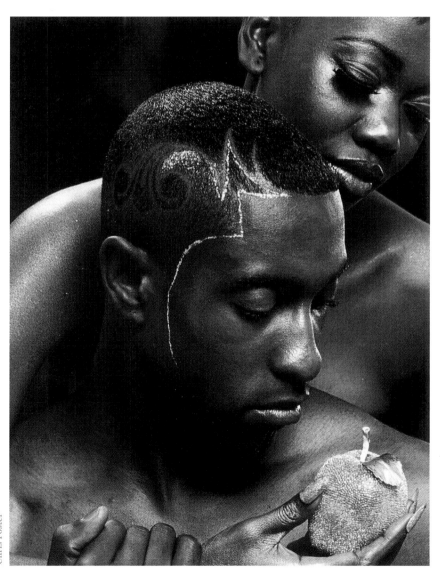

Chris Foster

Here are some important points to remember about outlining men's haircuts:

- On most men the haircut must be outlined or it will appear untidy and unfinished.
- Follow the natural hairline wherever possible, particularly when outlining short haircuts. Avoid making unnecessary cuts into the natural hairline, especially around the ears and at the sides of the nape. (Such cuts would appear harsh and unnatural, and the haircut would soon appear untidy when the hair started to grow back.)
- Many outlines, particularly on shorter styles, appear more natural if they are gently tapered in the nape and at the bottom of the sideburns.
- Some African-Caribbean men have outlines created at the front to add definition to their style.

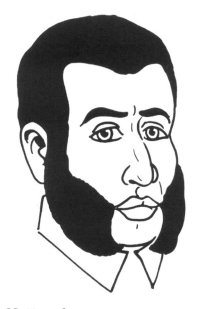

Mutton chops

Cutting sideburns

At one time most men wore a beard, a moustache, or long sideburns. The sideburns were often grown so long that they reached the bottom of the jawbone, and long distinctive sideburn shapes such as mutton chops became a prominent feature in men's fashion for many years. The introduction of the safety razor in about 1905 helped to establish the popularity of the clean-shaven appearance, and men started wearing their sideburns much shorter.

Today, sideburns are important in most men's haircuts, particularly on shorter styles because the sideburns are more visible. Many young men are now wearing longer sideburns, often shaped into points or other more elaborate designs. Most men, however, want sideburn shapes that are less prominent, with the emphasis on creating a natural, balanced look. The face shape and the hairstyle should be used to determine the correct choice of sideburn shape for each client.

Here are some important points to remember about cutting sideburns:

- Most men's haircuts are improved by having sideburns. When cut to the correct length sideburns help to balance the haircut and create an attractive, masculine frame to the face.
- Avoid cutting the length of the sideburns higher than the top of the ear and into the hairline, as this creates a particularly harsh and unnatural effect. Men sometimes do this inadvertently when shaving, so offer advice on how to avoid this (see the tip below and Chapter 11, 'Shaving'). A drop of about 2cm from the top of the ear is often acceptable, but remember to take into account other factors.
- Always ensure that the sideburns are cut level. Do not use the ears to determine the level of the sideburns, as they themselves are seldom level.

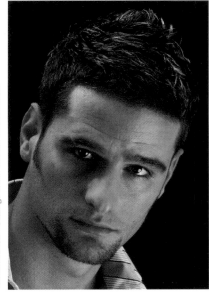

Tip

To ensure that the sideburns are cut level, place the thumb of each hand high on each sideburn. Whilst looking in the mirror, slide one thumb down until the desired length is reached. Slide the other thumb down until both thumbs are level. Memorise the position of the thumbs – you can note a position on each ear as a point of reference. Now cut each sideburn to the correct length.

Consider sharing this tip with your clients, many of whom may have difficulty keeping their sideburns level when shaving.

Further information on cutting sideburns and other facial hair is provided in Chapter 4, 'Cutting facial hair using basic techniques'.

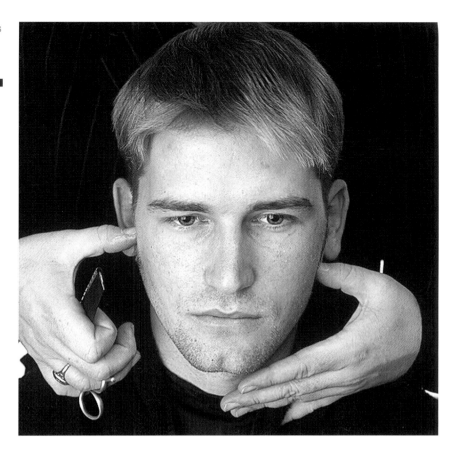

● Pay particular attention to where the haircut meets the sideburns and ensure that they blend together. You should think of these as being integrated parts of one style. Do not cut straight across the sideburns when outlining the haircut – this would produce a line across the sideburn through which the skin could be seen. The sideburns should be outlined by following down their natural hairline, adjacent to the ear.

Neckline shapes

The outline of the haircut in the nape is called the neckline shape. The neckline is important in men's hairdressing: the natural neck hairline is usually less well defined as hair often grows densely on the neck.

Over the years three basic neckline shapes have been developed to produce the looks that men like whilst ensuring that the haircut does not become untidy too quickly when the neck hair grows back. The three shapes are:

● **squared neckline shapes** These are sometimes known as a square cut.

● **tapered neckline shapes** These are sometimes known as a taper cut.

● **rounded neckline shapes** These are sometimes known as a Boston neckline.

A natural tapered neck

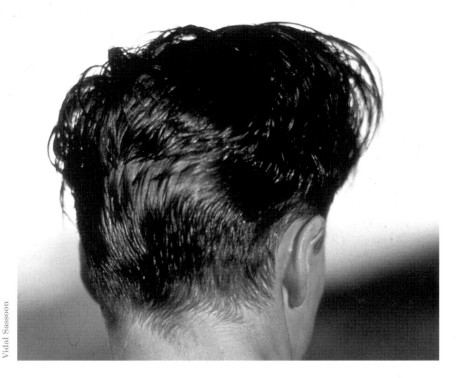

Vidal Sassoon

Squared neckline shapes

Squared neckline shapes have clean distinct outlines that form a square shape. They can be achieved with scissors or electric clippers, which are often inverted and used to cut the neckline straight across. The neckline should be cut into a square corner where it meets the outline at the sides of the nape.

These outlines must be cut to follow the natural hairline, or a true square-cut shape will not be produced. Do not make any cuts into these outlines, as they would appear harsh and unnatural and the removed hair would soon grow back to make the haircut appear untidy. If required, the square-cut neckline may be gently tapered to produce a softer, more natural finish.

Cutting a squared neckline

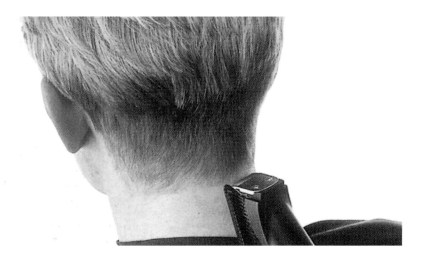

Simon Shaw

Tapered neckline shapes

Tapered neckline

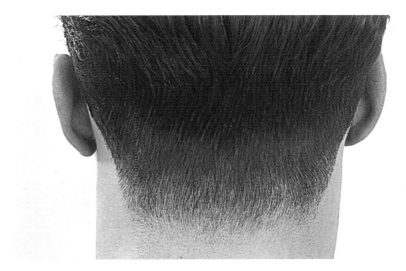

Tapered neckline shapes have soft, graduated outlines that follow the natural hairline in the nape. They are far less severe than a squared neckline. The hair may be graduated through most of the back and sides of the head, or it may just be applied to the last few centimetres of hair at the bottom of the nape. Tapered necklines are usually achieved with scissors-over-comb and clippers-over-comb cutting techniques, though clipper attachments can also be used.

As with squared necklines, it is important that the outlines at the sides of the nape are cut to follow the natural hairline. Indeed, the whole neckline shape should still appear square, but without any distinct outlines.

Rounded neckline shapes

Rounded neckline

Tip

Cut the *sides* of the nape outlines before cutting *across* the neckline. This will help you to judge the proportions of the head and neck more clearly, and so determine the correct height at which to cut the neckline.

When cutting necklines, remember to take into account any hair growth patterns in the nape such as nape whorls, and ensure that these do not distort the required shape.

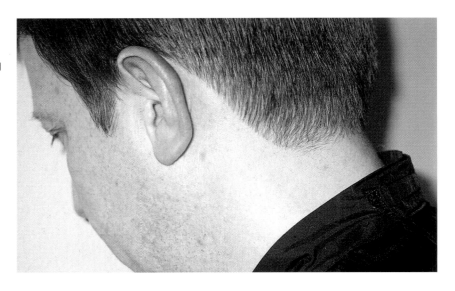

Rounded neckline shapes are similar to squared neckline shapes. They too have distinct outlines and appear square-shaped, but the corners of the neckline are then gently rounded. Rounded necklines can be achieved with scissors or electric clippers. Avoid making the shape too round, as rounded shapes are more feminine and are not usually suited to most men; also, any hair removed by such round shapes will soon grow back and make the haircut appear untidy. If required, rounded neckline shapes may be gently tapered to produce a softer, more natural finish.

Consultation prior to cutting men's hair

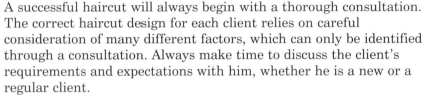

Health & Safety

A thorough consultation will ensure that you identify any adverse conditions of the hair or skin that may be present. It is particularly important to establish whether a suspected infection or infestation is present: this would prevent you from carrying out the shave. (This area is covered more fully in Chapter 2, 'Client care for men'.)

A successful haircut will always begin with a thorough consultation. The correct haircut design for each client relies on careful consideration of many different factors, which can only be identified through a consultation. Always make time to discuss the client's requirements and expectations with him, whether he is a new or a regular client.

Here are some of the critical factors you must consider when cutting men's hair.

- Identify the client's requirements, then give him advice on suitable styles. Agree the final effect to be achieved.
- Look for signs of broken skin or any abnormalities on the skin or hair.
- Look for signs of any unusual hair growth patterns, and identify the natural fall of the hair.
- Determine whether the hair is fine, medium or coarse.
- Is the hair growth dense or sparse? Does the client have male-pattern baldness?
- Is the client wearing an added hairpiece?
- Does the client have a beard or a moustache?
- Determine the features of the client's head, face and body. Is the client wearing spectacles or a hearing aid?
- Take into account the approximate age of the client.
- Consider the client's lifestyle.

Hair growth patterns

Hair growth patterns are the way in which individual hairs or a section of the hair may grow in a particular direction. Hair growth patterns must be identified because they determine both the looks that can be created and the techniques that you should use. Some clients have very strong hair growth patterns: these need careful attention to produce the best effects, and sometimes just to prevent the hair from sticking straight up!

Here are some unusual hair growth patterns and the most suitable ways of cutting them.

Double crown

With a double crown the hair is usually best left longer. If cut too short, the hair will stick up and will never lie flat.

A double crown

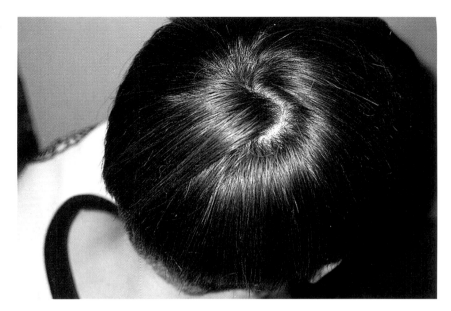

Nape whorl

A nape whorl

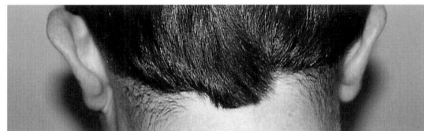

Dr John Gray

A nape whorl may be found at either side of the nape, and sometimes at *both* sides. It can make the hair difficult to cut into a straight neckline – often the hair naturally forms a V-shape. Tapered neckline shapes may be more suitable, but sometimes the hair is best left long so that the weight of the hair overcomes the nape whorl movement.

Cowlick

A cowlick

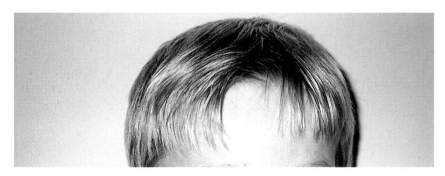

The cowlick is found on the hairline at the front of the head. It makes cutting a straight fringe difficult, particularly on fine hair, because the hair often forms a natural parting. It is usually better to cut the hair following this shape. Sometimes a fringe can be achieved by leaving the layers longer so that they weigh down the hair.

Widow's peak

A widow's peak

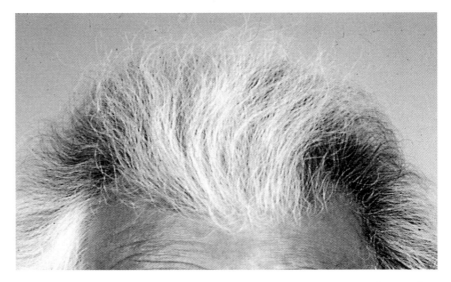

The widow's peak growth pattern appears at the front hairline. The hair grows upward and forward, forming a strong peak. It is usually better to cut the hair into styles that are dressed back from the face, as any fringe would be likely to separate and stick up. Short cropped styles or a parting may also be suitable, and sometimes a fringe is possible if the layers are left long.

Texture

The texture of hair can be fine, medium or coarse. Fine hair can be easy to cut, but some fuller styles will be more difficult to create and 'steps' are often more easily produced. Coarse hair can be more difficult to cut and is liable to fly in all directions during cutting, particularly on very short styles, so extra care must be taken to protect the client's and your own eyes. It is important when cutting very coarse hair to use sharp cutting tools and to take small cutting sections.

Type

Hair type may be tight curly, curly, wavy or straight. Each hair type must be considered because the different types will behave differently when cut, so particular cutting techniques are more suited to some types than others. Here are some examples.

- **Tight curly hair** Tight curly hair is often very difficult to cut with scissors-over-comb techniques, so scissors- or clippers-over-fingers and freehand cutting techniques are mostly used. Razor-cutting is not usually suitable.
- **Curly hair** Curly hair will coil back after being stretched during cutting, so remember not to cut it too short! Scissors- or clippers-over-comb techniques may be more difficult to use efficiently and accurately on curly hair, so cutting over the fingers is usually best.

- **Wavy hair** Any of the cutting techniques can be used with wavy hair, but the position of the waves requires careful attention. Careful cutting is needed to ensure that the resulting wave movement suits the required look. Cutting the crests of the waves too short can make the hair stick up: dressing the hair into shape would then be difficult.

- **Straight hair** Straight hair – and especially fine straight hair – requires small, accurate sections to be used or marks and 'steps' may become visible. Straight hair may be cut with any of the cutting techniques, but razor-cutting on fine hair is usually not required.

Density

Hair density is the amount of hair that grows in a given area of the scalp. It determines the choice of hairstyle that can be created and affects the techniques that are used.

Baldness

Many people experience a noticeable reduction in the density of their hair as they get older. Common baldness is the most frequent cause of this hair loss. It can affect both men and women, but it is much more common in men. Indeed, about 50 per cent of men experience some hair loss by the age of 50, so many men must accept the likelihood of going bald, especially if their fathers have lost their hair.

Most baldness in men is caused by male-pattern alopecia. This is a hereditary condition in which some hair follicles stop producing terminal hairs and revert to producing vellus-type hairs. It is thought to result from the influence of the male hormone called androgen. The affected follicles usually follow a distinct pattern, the Hamilton pattern (page 29), which is seen in men throughout the world.

The exact causes of male-pattern alopecia are still not fully understood, but over the years many different cures have been tried, usually with little success. Some men try to disguise the advanced

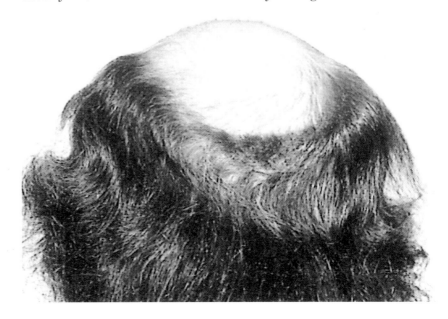

Tip

Before cutting the hair, especially with new clients, always look for signs of male-pattern alopecia or of alopecia areata: the hair may have been left long in some areas to cover the baldness. Cutting the hair too short in these areas would expose the skin, which would not go unnoticed!

Tip

The ends of the hair in the long hair section combed across the top of the head must be tapered and thinned to ensure that they blend in with the hair at the other side of the head. This is achieved with scissor tapering techniques applied to small sub-sections of the hair at a time. Use a slithering, backwards-and-forwards movement.

Take great care not to cut the hair too short, or it will no longer reach the hair on the other side and the scalp will become visible. Never just cut this section of hair straight across: if you did, a harsh line would be clearly visible.

stages of baldness by creating an unusually low parting in their remaining hair. The parted hair section is then grown long and combed up and over the bald area. This strategy is not particularly successful, as the section of hair may be many centimetres in length and is easily blown about when outdoors. Large amounts of sprays and dressings may be used to hold the hair in place, but the effect this creates is often unnatural and may simply cause the long strands of hair to be blown up together, exposing the scalp beneath and leading to considerable embarrassment.

On most bald men, short layered looks and leaner haircut shapes are usually more flattering. These looks are more natural and more manageable, although men are often anxious about 'going short' on the first occasion, especially if they usually have long hair.

The impact of baldness on men should not be underestimated. During the consultation, handle this subject with great care. Always respect the client's wishes, especially with men who wish to retain the style with a low parting or who wear added hairpieces.

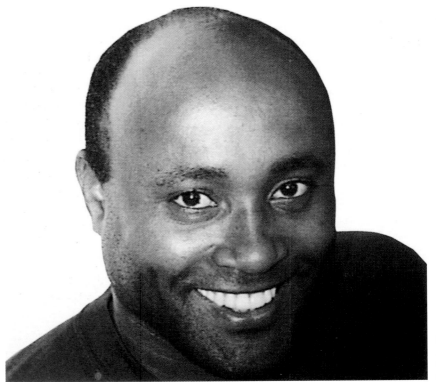

Dr John Gray

Added hairpieces

Some bald men wear added hairpieces because they prefer the look that these create. Cutting a new hairpiece into shape is a specialist service that should be attempted only by those competent in this type of work. Further studies will be necessary if you are interested in acquiring these skills.

Some barbers specialise in providing such services and establish long and profitable relationships with their clients, but often the manufacturer or supplier of the hairpiece carries out this work. However, any barber will benefit by being able to *recognise* that an established hairpiece is worn and by knowing how to cut the client's natural hair to suit.

Tip

If the client wears spectacles or an external hearing aid, ask him to remove them while you cut his hair, but remember to take them into account during cutting. Some spectacles may cause the hair to stick out if it is not cut correctly. Hearing aids often clip over the back of the ear, and the client may wish you to leave the hair longer to disguise this.

Tip

If the client has a beard or moustache you must think of these as being integrated parts of one style. Choose a haircut shape to suit the total look.

Here are some important things to remember about working with hairpieces.

- **Full hairpieces** Men who wear full hairpieces usually remove the hairpiece before visiting the barber's shop. They often have their natural hair cut short because it is not visible when the hairpiece is worn.

- **Smaller hairpieces and toupees** Some barbers leave smaller hairpieces and toupees in place while they cut the client's natural hair. The hairpiece hair is sectioned at the bottom and held out of the way with cutting clips to gain access to the natural hair beneath. (Do not use brightly coloured butterfly clips – these would certainly embarrass the client.) This method of cutting is sometimes preferable because it allows the barber to determine the correct length at which the natural hair should be cut and so blend the hairpiece in more effectively. Scissors-over-comb cutting techniques are used, and great care must be taken as any cuts to the hairpiece will not grow back!

- **Removing hairpieces** Hairpieces are usually held in place by special double-sided sticky tape. They should be removed by the client himself, to avoid causing any discomfort.

Features

The features of the client's head, face and body must all be noted to ensure that you choose the most suitable haircut shape. Every haircut should be designed to suit the head and face shape. Your decisions about the hair length, thickness and balance must all relate to the features of these underlying structures.

Careful consideration must be given to each of the following:

- the shape of the face – round, square, oblong, long, short, or whatever
- the size and position of the ears
- the size and shape of the nose
- the shape of the jaw and chin
- any unusual features, such as a high front hairline
- the way the head and body are held
- the length and width of the neck

Different head and face shapes require different haircut shapes. Here are some examples.

- **a round face** Choose a haircut shape that is dressed higher at the front and top. The sides should be less full, or leaner. Avoid full, round shapes, as they would make the face appear more round.

- **a large head and face** A large, full haircut shape may be more suitable, as a small shape can appear lost and out of proportion, but the shape of the face must also be considered.

- **a small head and face** The smaller face is more suited to less full, leaner haircut shapes: the face would appear swamped by large, full and fussy styles.

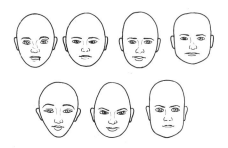

Face and head shapes

- **a large nose** Fuller shapes with side partings usually help to diminish a large nose. Avoid centre partings and dressing the hair straight back off the forehead.
- **a tall person** Taller shapes accentuate the person's height, so flatter shapes are better.
- **a short person** Flatter shapes will make short people appear shorter, so taller shapes are usually best.
- **a long face** Choose a shape that is fuller at the sides and shorter on the top. This will help to make the face appear less long.
- **a square face** Taller shapes are often more suitable. They should be short and less full at the sides, but longer and higher towards the top.
- **an oval face** An oval face shape is considered to be the ideal because most haircut shapes will suit it. Remember to take into account the client's other features, however, such as the position of his eyes and ears.

Age

The client's age must be considered because people of different ages usually require different hairstyles.

- **Children** Children mostly require simple hairstyles that need little or no dressing and styling, so shorter styles are often best.
- **Teenagers** Teenagers wear many different styles. Some of these are common to older age groups, but many young men want highly personalised styles. This age group is often prepared to carry out daily grooming, blow-styling and dressing to achieve their chosen look. Distinctive and sometimes quite extreme looks are required, which may be either short or long.

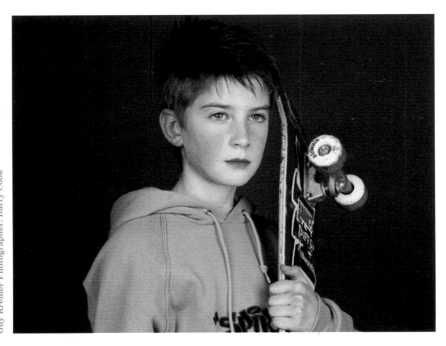

Guy Kremer Photographer: Barry Cook

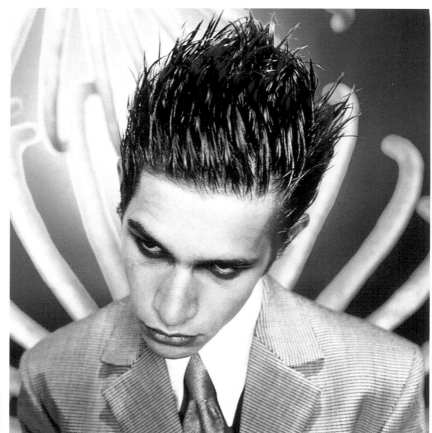

Danial Hill

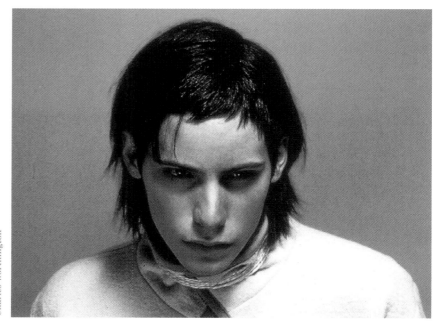

Charles Worthington

● **Young men** Young men usually require fashionable but practical styles which are easy to manage and are in keeping with their chosen style of clothing. Preferred styles are often similar to those worn by teenagers, but usually less extreme.

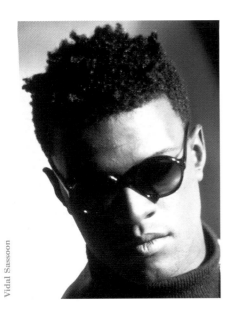

Vidal Sassoon

- **Mature men** Mature men usually require practical styles that are easy to maintain. Shorter shapes are most popular.

Lifestyle

The client's lifestyle also affects the choice of haircut design. Busy men may not have the time to look after fussy styles; long hair may not be suitable for those who take part in a lot of sport, as drying the hair can take too long. Particular jobs sometimes require particular haircuts – for example, short haircuts are required for those in the army, fire service or police.

Tools and equipment

Tools

All haircutting tools must be well-balanced, sharp, clean and safe to use. Here are the main tools required for cutting men's hair.

Scissors

Scissors are available in different sizes, ranging from 10cm to 18cm. Barbers usually prefer scissors around 15cm in length, but it depends on what feels comfortable in the size of your hand and for the job you are doing.

Tip

Do not let other barbers use your scissors. They become accustomed to your grip and can become blunt more quickly if used by others.

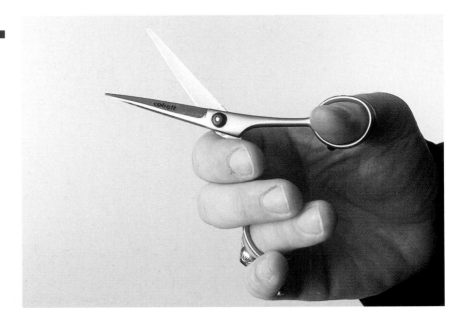

Haircutting scissors should be held with the thumb through one handle and the third finger through the other. Only the blade that is operated by the thumb should move when the scissors are being used. This method will produce the most accurate results and it provides the most control and stability, which is vital when cutting around delicate areas such as the ears.

 Tip

Develop your skills by using the scissors before you start cutting any hair. A good exercise is to open and close the scissors several times whilst moving up along a flat vertical surface. Concentrate on making the thumb blade move whilst keeping the other blade still. Make the movements slowly at first – increase the speed only when you become more proficient.

 Tip

Ensure scissors are always kept sharp by using professional sharpening services.

Good-quality hairdressing scissors can be quite expensive, but they will last you for many years if you look after them. Only ever use them for cutting hair, or they will quickly become blunt. Keep them clean, and always remove loose hairs, grease and any dirt before disinfecting or sterilising them. Never use dirty scissors because of the risk of passing infection from one client to another.

Clean and lubricate the scissors regularly, and especially before using them on each new client. Many different disinfectants, alcohol wipes and disinfectant sprays are available for this purpose.

Thinning scissors are used to remove bulk without removing length. The blades are serrated so that when the blades are closed only some of the hairs are cut. One or both of the blades may be serrated,

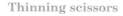
Thinning scissors

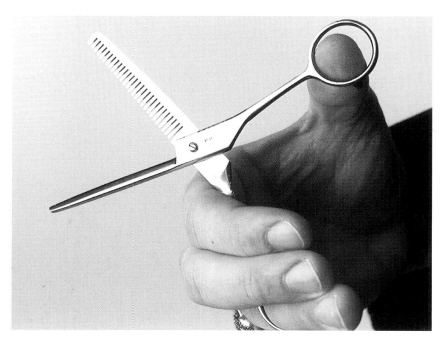

and scissors are available with different numbers and sizes of serrations. The size and number of the serrations determine how many hairs are cut when the blades are closed.

Clippers

Clippers may be either hand-operated or electric. Hand clippers are operated by squeezing the handles together. They are seldom used today unless there is no access to electricity, such as during a power cut. Electric clippers or trimmers may be powered by either mains electricity or rechargeable batteries, and are operated by an electric motor or a magnetic coil.

Electric clippers are the preferred choice today because of their power, accuracy and convenience in comparison with hand clippers. They are available in three different designs:

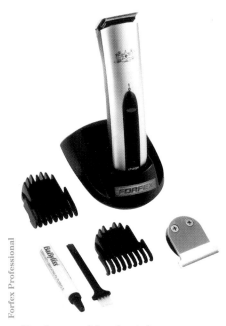

Forfex Professional

Rechargeable electric trimmers with detachable blades

Tip

Make sure that you change detachable blades over a working surface to avoid them dropping to the floor and being damaged.

- **Detachable-blade electric clippers** These have a wide range of blade sizes available and tend to be operated by powerful electric motors, making them suitable for all types of work. The blades are easily changed, as the new selected blade is simply pushed on to the clipper head when required. The blades are quite delicate though and must be handled carefully to avoid dropping them. Detachable-blade clippers are easy to clean. The blades and a blade storage box can usually be purchased separately if not provided with the clippers.

- **Adjustable-blade electric clippers** Adjustable-blade clippers are very versatile, as the blades can be set across a wide range of cutting depths, although the range does not usually cut quite as close as the closest cutting detachable blade. Adjustable-blade clippers are preferred by many barbers, as they are self-contained and the barber does not need to carry additional blades. This makes them easy to transport and very suitable for freelance work. They are usually operated by a magnetic coil, which means they are quieter and therefore less frightening for smaller children. The blades can be easily dismantled for cleaning. Some adjustable-blade electric clippers now have predetermined depth settings to make it easier to select a specific cutting depth, helping the barber work consistently.

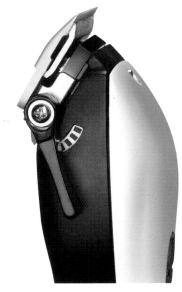

Forfex Professional

Adjustable-blade electric trimmers

Tip

A wide range of accessories is available for all types of clippers and trimmers, including:

- detachable comb attachments
- storage units
- charging units (where relevant)
- cleaning equipment and products
- lubricants

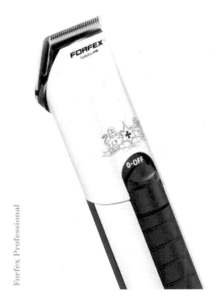

Non-adjustable blade trimmers

Tip

Some clippers are now fitted with ceramic blades that should never need sharpening.

● **Non-detachable-blade electric clippers/trimmers**
Non-detachable-blade electric clippers or trimmers, as they are often called, are mostly used for outlining haircuts and facial hair shapes, especially around the lips, and for cleaning hair from the nape. Indeed, they are sometimes used to remove hair from the nape area in women's hairdressing. They are usually smaller than detachable-blade and adjustable-blade clippers and so are easier to use in confined areas, such as under the nose. Closer cutting blades are usually fitted and units are normally operated by less powerful electric motors or magnetic coils. The blades can usually be dismantled for cleaning.

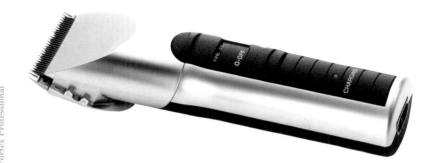

Rechargeable ceramic blade clippers

Clippers are equipped with a range of different blade sizes for different purposes. The number 000 blade is good for removing hair from outside the outlines, whilst the number 1 blade is best for clipper-cutting the hair to remove bulk.

Here are the most common sizes available.

	Blade sizes	*Cutting length of blade*
Detachable blades The blades are available in a wide range of sizes.	0000 000 00 0 0A 1 1A 11/2 2 3	A very close cut (similar to shaving) 0.3mm (a close cut) 0.4mm 0.8mm 1.2mm 3.3mm 4.0mm 4.8mm 6.4mm 7.9mm
Adjustable blade Moving a small lever alters the cutting length of the blade. (Hand-operated clippers often have adjustable blades.)	From 000 to 1	As above
Non-adjustable blade	A fixed setting between 000 and 1	As above

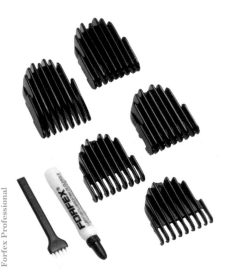

Forfex Professional

Texturising and razoring blades

Recently detachable texturising blades and razoring blades have become available for some clippers. The cutting edge of texturising blades resembles castellated scissors. They have preset gaps in the guard so that more hair is removed in just these areas in order to produce different textured effects within the haircut. Razoring blades too can produce textured effects but these mainly give results similar to traditional razoring.

Detachable comb attachments are also available for electric clippers, which give a wide range of predetermined cutting lengths. These allow for very fast removal of hair and are sometimes used to reduce the length of the hair and produce a rough shape, which is then finished with scissors and clippers (without the comb attached). The combs are available in sizes ranging from a number 8, which will leave the hair about 25mm long, to a number 1, which will leave the hair only about 1mm long after cutting. The most popular sizes are the number 3, which leaves the hair about 10mm long, and the number 4, which leaves the hair about 13mm long.

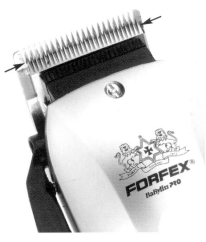

Forfex Professional

![!]

Health & Safety

Before using the clippers, and especially after cleaning the blades, always check that the top, movable cutting blade is not protruding beyond the lower, static blade. If the movable blade protrudes it would cut the client's skin.

Razors

Razors are used in men's haircutting to shave outlines, to thin and style the hair, or to produce textured effects. Disposable-blade razors are preferable because they are more hygienic. Detailed information on razors is provided in Chapter 11, 'Shaving'.

Combs

Combs are available in various different sizes for different purposes. Cutting combs are usually thin and pliable, with fine teeth at one side and coarse teeth at the other. The coarse teeth should be used for most combing and sectioning, while the fine teeth are good for detailed work and close cutting. The barber comb is specifically designed for this purpose. It is very thin and pliable and the side with the fine teeth narrows to a point. This makes the comb easier to use when producing fine tapered finishes, especially in confined areas, such as around the ears.

A cutting comb should fit comfortably in the hand and be easy to move into all the positions required during cutting.

Forfex Professional

Checking alignment of the cutting blade

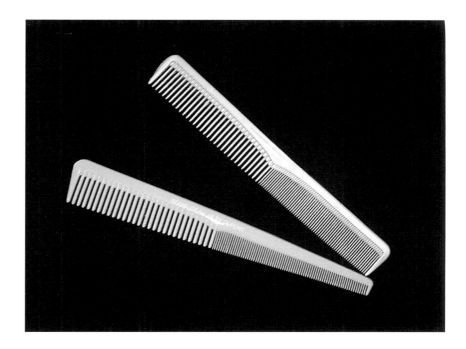

Neck brush

A neck brush is required to remove excess hair cuttings and to maintain the client's comfort throughout the service.

Equipment

The client should be seated in an adjustable chair (see page 207), which can be positioned at the correct height so that the hair can be worked on efficiently.

Preparation for cutting hair

1   Carry out your consultation with the client.

2   Determine the client's wishes and confirm what is to be done. Use photographs or pictures to help clarify the required shape.

3   Before you begin work, gather together all the tools and equipment you will require.

4   Gown the client, placing a clean tissue or neckstrip between the client's neck and the gown. A cutting collar may then be placed on top of the gown. Some barbers use a clean towel instead of a cutting collar, particularly if the hair is wet. This should be placed across the client's back and be tucked in at the neck.

5   Position the client in a chair so that the hair can be worked on efficiently.

6   Carefully comb the hair, disentangling it if required. Look out for areas of sparse growth, scarring or other unusual features you may not have seen earlier.

Basic cutting techniques

The techniques used for cutting men's hair are generally the same as those used in women's hairdressing. The barber understands, however, that differences exist in the way the techniques are used and in the effects they achieve.

The following cutting techniques are commonly used when cutting men's hair.

Club cutting

In club cutting the sections of the hair are cut straight across to produce blunt ends which are all cut at the same length. Small sections are required, particularly on coarse, dense hair, or the hair ends will not be level. This technique may be used on wet or dry hair.

Here are the main methods of club cutting used in men's hairdressing.

Scissors-over-comb

Scissors-over-comb technique

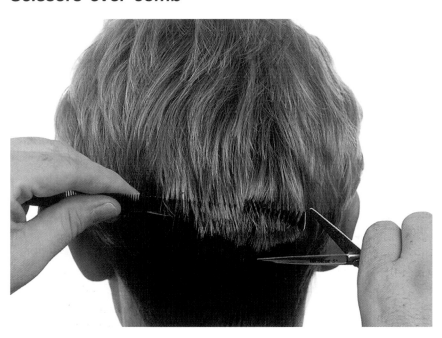

Tip

Make sure that your scissors are fully closed before using the tips to lift sections of hair when doing scissors-over-comb or the open blade will snag the hair and cut it short near the roots.

The scissors-over-comb technique is performed by lifting a section of hair and then cutting it straight across. When cutting short hairs in the nape you should take extra-small sections of hair, which are usually lifted with the comb. Some barbers use the tips of their scissors to lift the longer sections of hair, which are then picked up on the comb and positioned ready for cutting. Ensure that you use the coarse teeth of the comb and the main part of the scissors when cutting the interior of the haircut, and the fine teeth and the tips of the scissors when working around the ears and nape.

Scissors-over-comb is mostly used on shorter styles, particularly to create graduation in the nape and at the sides.

Clubbing over the fingers

Clubbing over the fingers

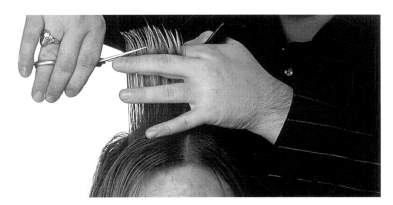

Clubbing over the fingers is very similar to the scissors-over-comb technique – indeed, it might be called 'scissors-over-fingers'. It is performed by lifting a section of the hair, which is then combed out and transferred to the fingers. The fingers slide up the section of hair to the correct position for cutting, and the hair is then cut straight across. The hair may be held at different angles, and different sizes of sections may be used, to create the amount of graduation required.

Clubbing over the fingers is mostly used on longer styles and to cut the top of many short styles.

Clippers-over-comb

Clippers-over-comb technique

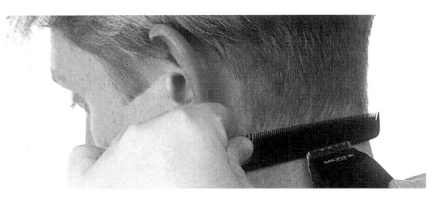

Clippers-over-comb can be used instead of scissors-over-comb and clubbing-over-the-fingers techniques, especially on long, coarse and dense hair, and particularly if it is being taken much shorter. Many of the same effects possible with scissors can also be achieved using clippers. Clippers are best used on dry hair.

Freehand cutting

Freehand cutting is the cutting of hair without first taking the hair into a section or holding the hair in place with the comb or hand. It is often used to remove individual hairs or small amounts of hair when finishing a style, or for producing textured effects. It is usually performed with the tips of the scissors.

Freehand cutting can be particularly useful when cutting tight curly or curly hair, and is often used on beards and moustaches to smooth the outline shape and remove stray hairs. Tapered effects can also be achieved freehand by using sliding and slicing movements.

Tight curly hair

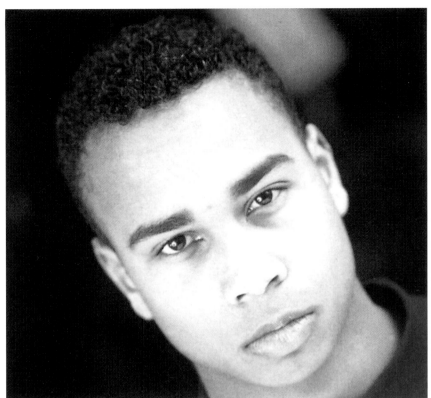

Ralph Kleeli

Thinning

Thinning techniques are used to remove bulk and thickness without affecting the overall length. Thinning is achieved by cutting just *some* of the hairs in a section of hair, while leaving others uncut so that the length of the overall section remains unchanged. The hair should be cut only in the middle third of the section: if it is cut too close to the roots, the resulting short hairs will stick straight out.

Here are the most common methods used for thinning men's hair.

Scissor thinning

Scissor thinning or point cutting

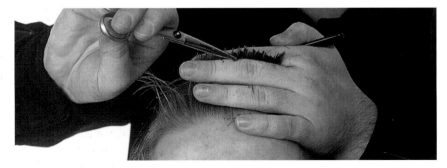

Scissor thinning is achieved using a similar action to that used in scissor tapering, but here the open scissor blades are moved along the hair section in one long movement. The hair may also be cut with the points of the scissors, known as point cutting or pointing – this technique should be used in the middle of the hair section. Sometimes it is used to thin the ends of the hair and to create softer lines.

Cutting with thinning scissors

Cutting with thinning scissors

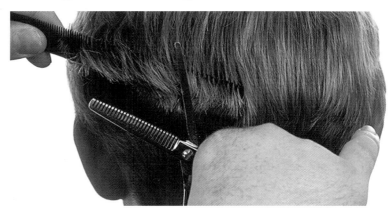

Thinning scissors have serrated blades: when closed, they cut only some of the hairs. They should be used in the middle third of the section or towards the ends.

Thinning with a razor

Thinning with a razor

Tip

Take great care when cutting with a razor. Do not razor-cut the hair too near to the hairline or roots.

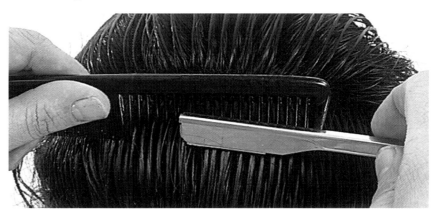

Thinning with a razor is carried out only on wet hair. It is achieved by placing the razor on the hair at an angle of about 30–40° and then cutting the hair by gentle slicing movements. Gentle actions are required or the hair will be cut straight through!

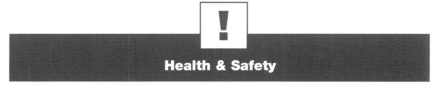

Health & Safety

Razors have very sharp blades and must always be treated with care and respect. Keep the handle closed or cover the blade when not in use, and especially when carrying or passing a razor. Never place a razor in your pockets, and always keep razors out of the reach of children.

Skin fading

Skin fading is the term used mostly in African-Caribbean hairdressing to describe very close short graduation with clippers that leaves no visible outline at the back and sides – the hair simply appears to *fade* into the skin. The cut increases from a 0000 sized detachable blade or 000 adjustable blade setting in the nape and around the ears up to a length of several centimetres on the top.

Partings and fringes

Partings

Many men's hairstyles have partings. These can be used in many different ways and to create many different effects. For example, partings may be used to draw attention away from unwanted prominent facial features, such as a large nose or large ears. Centre partings and side partings are often used to divide large hair masses and produce more pleasing and symmetrical shapes, which are also more manageable.

Many men have natural partings. To identify these, comb the wet hair straight back, then push it forward with the palm of the hand: where the hair parts naturally is the natural parting. Such partings should be used, where possible, as the resulting style will be easier to manage. The natural hair growth patterns and the hair fall must all be identified and considered to determine where, if at all, a parting is required.

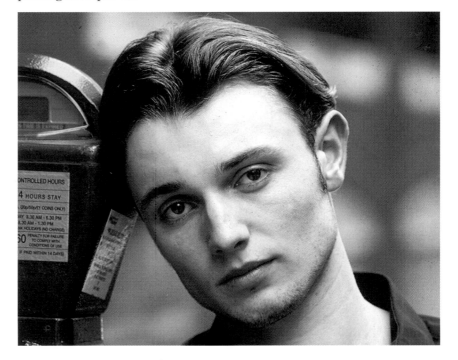

Fringes

The front of the hair may be dressed into a fringe. Men do not often wear full fringes, but many children do. A fringe shape may be short, long, squared, rounded, blunt-cut or tapered.

The client's head and face shape will determine which fringe shape is best. The fringe should not be too heavy or it will appear

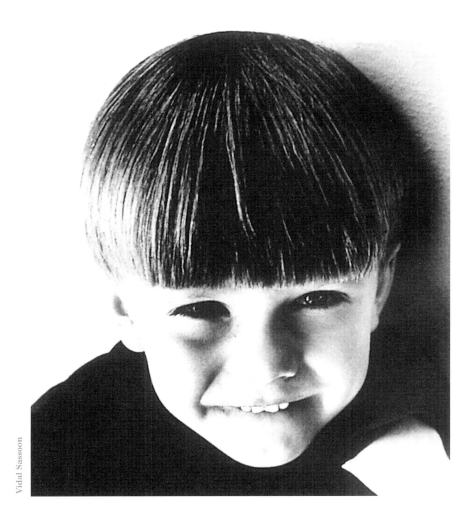

Vidal Sassoon

Tip

If you wish to carry out dry cutting, it is best to wash and dry the hair first. Be sure to explain this to the client first and take his wishes into account.

Tip

Remember that hair stretches by up to half its own length when wet. Keep this in mind when you are cutting stretched hair, so that it is not too short when it dries.

unnatural, and fringes can even look like artificial hair! Layering is often used to reduce the thickness, and the ends are sometimes tapered to produce a softer line. Hair growth patterns such as a cowlick or widow's peak must be considered as they may make a full fringe impractical. Remember that it is usually better to go *with* the natural hair fall rather than *against* it.

Wet and dry cutting

Traditionally, most men visited the barbers' shop to have their hair cut dry. A dry cut produced good results and was completed more quickly than a wet cut. Today, many men have their hair washed and then cut wet, but dry cutting is still common.

If the client's hair is greasy and dirty then it must be washed before you can cut it. Wet hair is also required for blow-styling and some cutting techniques, such as razor-cutting, which should always be carried out on wet hair to avoid causing damage to the hair and discomfort to the client. Other cutting techniques are less suitable for use on wet hair, such as some scissor-tapering and clippers-over-comb movements. In general, *scissors* can be used on wet or dry hair, razors must only be used on wet hair, and *thinning scissors* and *clippers* are best used on dry hair.

Layering

The purpose of layering is to produce a series of connected, unbroken layers, with no perceptible lines or 'steps' in between. Most men wear layered haircuts: these often produce a more masculine shape and are easier to manage.

Here are the two main layered effects that are mostly required in men's hairdressing.

Uniform layering

Uniform layering

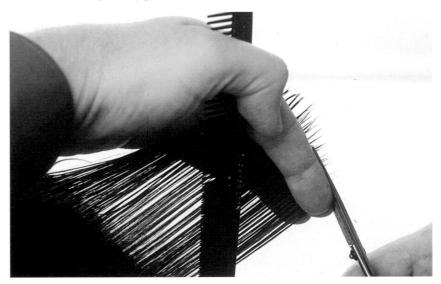

Uniform layering is the process of cutting the sections of the hair to the same length. It can be achieved by holding each section at 90° to the head, and then cutting the hair straight across at the same angle.

Uniform layering is used mostly in longer styles, and to cut the hair on the top of the head in some shorter styles. It is particularly suitable for creating shapes on curly hair.

Graduated layering

Graduated layering

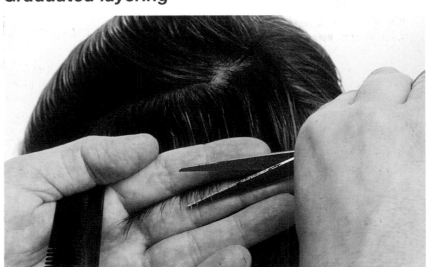

Graduated layering is the process of producing a difference in length between the layers at the top and the layers at the bottom of a section of hair. This can be achieved by elevating the sections of the hair at different angles and then cutting them straight through, or by holding the sections at 90° to the head and then cutting through the section at a different angle. Lifting the sections *higher* and then cutting them will produce a *greater* amount of graduation; holding them *lower* and then cutting will produce *less*.

The gradient between the top and bottom of the hair sections when positioned back on the head is called the angle of graduation.

- If you hold a section of hair at 90° (a right angle) to the back of the head, and cut it at 90° to the section, you will produce a 45° angle of graduation.
- If you hold a section of hair at 90° and cut it at 45° you will produce a steeper graduation.
- If you hold a section of hair at 90° and cut it at 145° you will produce a level length, in which all of the ends of the hair fall level, without graduation.

Many men's haircuts are graduated at the back and sides to produce taller, leaner, more masculine shapes.

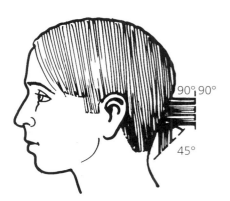

Producing a 45° angle of graduation

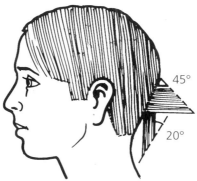

Producing a 20° angle of graduation

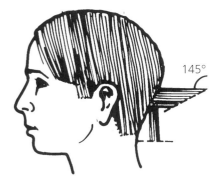

Producing a level length

Cutting guidelines

The cutting guideline is the line that is created by the ends of the hair when a section of hair is held out from the head. Establishing correct guidelines is very important when cutting the hair: if this is not done, the results will be uneven and inaccurate, and will not be likely to meet the client's requirements.

Some cutting guidelines are called the baseline or perimeter line. These are used to determine the outer and inner perimeters of the haircut. These lines are important because they usually provide the basis for the other guidelines to follow.

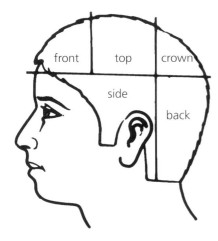

Guide section

To produce precise, accurate results, the guidelines should be carefully followed throughout the cutting process. Make sure that a guideline from a previously cut section of hair is clearly visible before cutting the new section of hair. Both the hair length and the line of the cut in the previous section should be used to guide where the next cut is to be made.

When preparing guidelines, many different factors must be considered – the position of the ears, the nose and the eyes, the shape of the head and the position of the hairlines, and so on. During the cutting process the head is often divided into large sections, rows or panels, to ensure that the guidelines are easily seen and to make the hair more manageable. Each of these sections or panels is then sub-divided into sections of hair for cutting. The cutting guideline established in one section is transferred from section to section, and panel to panel, so that the resulting haircut is connected throughout to produce an even result.

In men's hairdressing, particularly on shorter styles, the head is often divided into three main areas, which reflect the different shapes that are required and the techniques that are used.

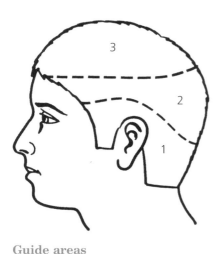

Guide areas

- Area 1 includes the hairline, the ear outline and the occipital bone. This is where most of the graduation and tapering is carried out. Usually scissors- or clippers-over-comb techniques are required.

- Area 2 is between the occipital bone and the bottom of the crown area. On shorter styles this is where the graduation and taper are blended into the hair in the top section. Thickness is often reduced here to create the taller, less full, more masculine shapes that most men prefer. Usually scissors- or clippers-over-comb and over-fingers techniques are required.

- Area 3 covers the rest of the top of the head, starting from the crown area. The blending of area 2 continues, and the lengths of the top and front are determined. Scissors- or clippers-over-comb cutting techniques can be used, but more often scissors- or clippers-over-fingers techniques are required.

Cutting procedures

In cutting men's hair, several different cutting procedures may be followed. Each individual barber will decide where to start and which cutting techniques to use, mainly according to personal preference.

Many different cutting techniques can achieve similar effects. They can also be combined and adapted as necessary, to achieve the required results. The best procedure is one that allows the barber to work accurately and efficiently throughout the whole haircut.

The following examples show how some common men's looks can be achieved using basic techniques.

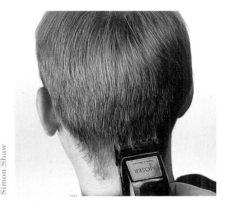

(a) Before cutting

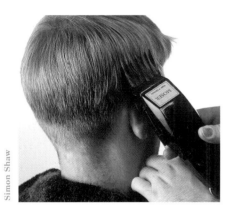

(b) Starting at the back

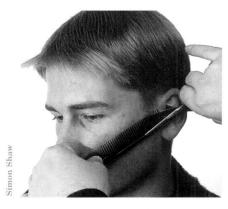

(c) Cutting the sides

(d) Shaping the sideburns

Short layered looks

Short graduation with a tapered neckline

1 Protect the client's clothes.

2 Comb the hair carefully, disentangling it where required (a).

3 Start in the centre panel of hair at the back of the head and begin cutting the hair (b). If using the clippers, choose the comb attachment for the length of cut you require. (The best size of comb for this look is either a number 3 or a number 4.) Ensure that the comb is securely attached to the clippers. A scissors- or clippers-over-comb technique may be used instead, if preferred.

4 Place the clippers flat against the neck, just below the neckline. Using a *smooth continuous movement*, push the clippers slowly up the head, keeping them flat against the scalp until you reach the area where you want the taper to begin. In a smooth *rocking* movement, *pivot* the clippers away from the head to produce the shape and length of hair that you want. Unless the top panels are to be cut short as well, *do not go higher than the occipital bone* without pivoting away from the head.

5 Move to the adjacent panel of hair and repeat the process as before. Make sure you follow the cutting guideline from the previous section and the adjacent panel. If the panels are not connected, long hairs will be left between them.

6 Keep working around the head, cutting the hair to the length determined by the chosen haircut shape. Do not cut the sides at this stage, if the hair is to be longer around the ears. Gradually increase the length of the hair by pivoting the clippers away as you work towards the sides (c).

7 Repeat this on the other side. As the shape develops, keep looking in the mirror to make sure that it is symmetrical. Consult with your client at regular intervals to confirm that the developing shape is correct, making adjustments if required.

8 Remove the comb attachment from the clippers. Move back to the centre panel of hair at the back of the head. Using either scissors- or clippers-over-comb techniques, begin to blend the hair where the top of the taper meets the hair on the top of the head. Move across the head, taking small sections. Ensure that the panels are connected, blending areas together to create an even, continuous effect.

9 Move to one side of the head. If your client has sideburns, note the required length. Carefully outline the sideburn and the hair around the ears (d, e), then move down the sides of the nape with the tips of your scissors or with the clippers. Use the fingers of your other hand to guide and support the scissors or clippers whilst cutting.

10 Repeat this on the other side of the head. Ensure that the sideburns are level (f: see the tip on page 68). As you create the outlines, *make sure you do not cut into the natural hairline, particularly at the sides of the nape* (g).

11 Position the client's head so that it is bent forward slightly. Carefully cut the neckline to the correct height. Use the

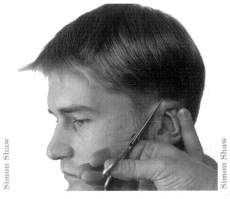

(e) Outlining hair around the ears

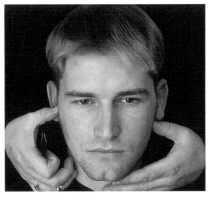

(f) Levelling the sideburns

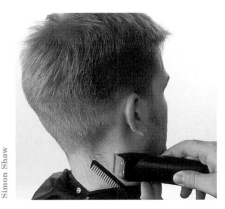

(g) Outlining the nape

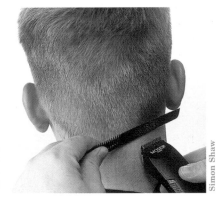

(h) Tapering around the neckline

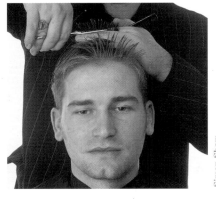

(i) Taking a section at the crown

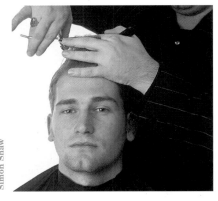

(j) Clubbing the top

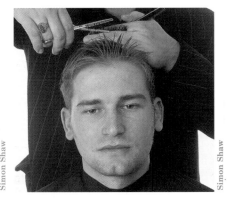

(k) Clubbing the top

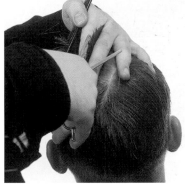

(l) Blending the top with the sides and back

proportions of the head and neck, the length of the hair and the position of the ears to determine the length that is most suitable. The neckline must be tapered to create a natural effect: do not cut it straight across. Use scissors-over-comb or clippers-over-comb techniques. The bottom edge of the comb should be held against the skin, then angled so that the hair will be cut shorter at the bottom and left longer at the top (h).

Tip

Before cutting the hair, make sure that you can clearly see the cutting guideline created by the previous section. If the hair is too thick for you to see the guideline through it, you may need to take a thinner section.

12 Move to the top of the head and take a section of hair at the crown (i). Using the clubbing-over-fingers technique, with either the scissors or clippers, cut the hair to the required length. Move across the head, taking small sections, and ensuring that successive panels of hair are connected, as before (j).

13 Blend the top panels and the side and back panels where they meet, to create an even, continuous effect.

14 Thinning techniques may be used through the top, as required (k, l).

15 Shave the areas outside the haircut outlines, if necessary (see Chapter 11, 'Shaving').

16 Graduate the outlines to blend them with the skin, where required.

17 Finish the shape by combing, styling and dressing the hair into place (m).

(m) The finished look

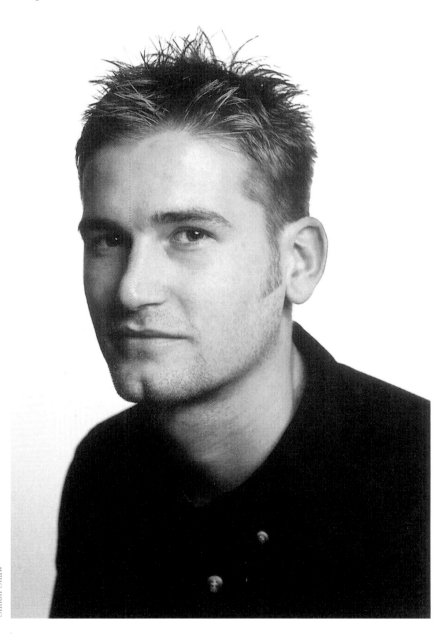

Simon Shaw

Short graduation, tapered neckline and razor thinning

A tapered neckline (without a detachable comb clipper attachment).

1 Protect the client's clothes.

2 Comb the hair carefully, disentangling where required.

3 With the hair wet, section the hair in two by making a parting from ear to ear across the top of the head and then a parting from this to the front. Take a section parallel to this parting at the crown and hold it at 90° to the head. Cut this section straight across to the correct length using the scissors-over-fingers technique.

4 Take a section going down the centre panel towards the front hairline and hold it at 90° to the head then cut this to the guideline from the first section. Continue down this panel to extend this guideline through the top (b).

5 Take the front section forwards and hold it at 90° then cut it to the required length for the front area.

6 Return to the crown area and take a small section parallel to the first parting and hold it at 90° to the head then cut it to length following the guideline from the first section. Continue working forward down the centre panel always cutting to the guideline from the previous section.

7 Move to the adjacent panel of hair and repeat the process making sure that the panels are connected.

8 Keep working around the top of the head cutting the hair to the length determined by the chosen haircut shape (c).

9 Make sure that the hair is still wet then begin thinning the hair through the top with the razor, following the panels used earlier. This will also help produce texture (d).

10 As the shape develops keep looking in the mirror to make sure that it is symmetrical. Consult with your client at regular intervals to confirm that the developing shape is correct, making adjustments if required.

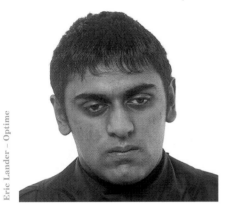

(a) Before cutting

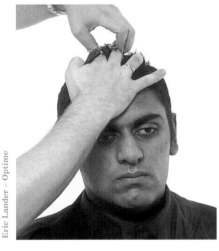

(b) Cutting the first guideline

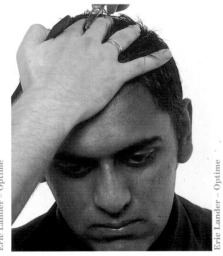

(c) Cutting the top

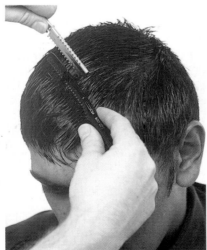

(d) Thinning with the razor

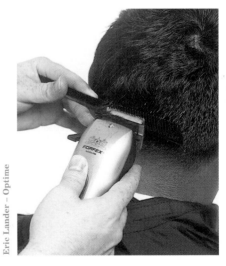

(e) Working across the back

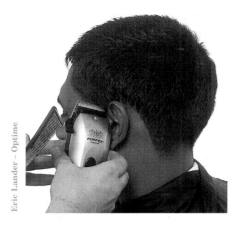

(f) **Outlining the sideburns**

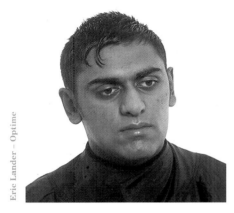

(g) **Styling and dressing**

11 Roughly dry the hair and move one side and begin cutting the hair to the required length using the clipper-over-comb technique. The hair length should be graduated to remove weight near the outline.

12 Move to the adjacent panel of hair and repeat the process, as before towards the middle of the nape. Make sure the panels are connected or long hairs will be left between each panel.

13 When the back is complete, move on to the other side of the head and continue cutting to the guideline.

14 Note the required length for any sideburns that may be present, ensure they are level (see tip on page 68) and cut them to shape. Carefully outline the sideburn and around the ears then down the sides of the nape with the edge of the clippers. Use the fingers of your other hand to guide and support the clippers whilst cutting.

15 Repeat this on the other side of the head. *Make sure you do not cut into the natural hairline when creating the outlines, particularly at the sides of the nape.*

16 Dry the hair into style.

17 Return to the centre panel of hair at the back of the head and finish the nape area, the neckline and the side outlines with the clippers-over-comb technique.

18 Use the proportions of the head and neck, the length of the hair and the position of the ears to determine the length that is most suitable. The neckline should be gently tapered to create a softer blended effect. The corners may be rounded, if required to produce a Boston neckline.

19 Shave the areas outside the haircut outlines, if required (see Chapter 11, 'Shaving').

20 Graduate the outlines to blend them with the skin, where required.

21 Finish the shape by combing, styling and dressing the hair into place (h).

(h) **The finished look**

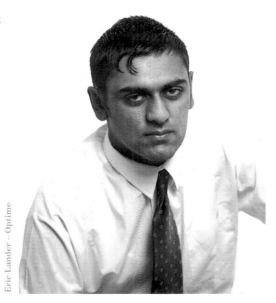

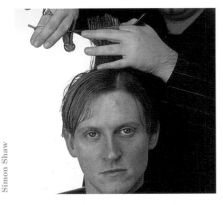

(a) **Before cutting**

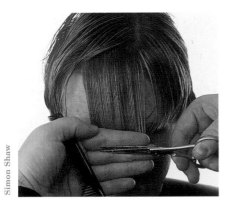

(b) **Cutting a section at the crown**

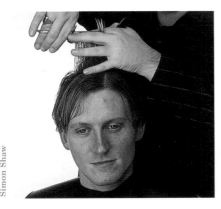

(c) **Cutting the front**

(d) **Cutting the centre panel**

Uniform layered top with a squared or rounded neckline

The procedure described is for a squared neckline. For a rounded neckline, follow this sequence and after the squared shape has been created, simply round off the corners of the neckline.

1 Protect the client's clothes.

2 Comb the hair carefully, disentangling it where required (a).

3 With the hair wet, section the hair in two by making a parting from ear to ear across the top of the head. Take a section *parallel* to this parting at the crown and hold it at 90° to the head (b). Cut this section straight across to the correct length using the scissors-over-fingers technique.

4 Take a section going down the centre panel towards the front hairline. Hold it at 90° to the head, then cut it to the guideline from the first section. Continue down this panel to extend this guideline through the top.

5 Take the front section forwards and hold it at 90°, then cut it to the required length for the front area. Remember: wet hair stretches, so do not cut it too short (c).

6 Return to the crown area. Take a small section, parallel to the first parting, and hold it at 90° to the head. Cut it to length, following the guideline from the first section. Continue working forward down the centre panel, always cutting to the guideline from the previous section (d).

7 Move to an adjacent panel of hair and repeat the process, making sure that the panels are connected.

8 Keep working around the top of the head, cutting the hair to the length determined by the chosen haircut shape.

9 Transfer the guideline down onto the side of the head by taking a vertical section. Continue cutting the sections through the sides to the required length. The hair length may be graduated to remove weight around the ears, if required, by angling the cut across the section.

10 As the shape develops, keep looking in the mirror to make sure that the shape is symmetrical. Consult with your client at regular intervals to confirm that the developing shape is correct, making adjustments if required.

11 Move to the crown area and transfer the guideline from the front of the first parting through to the back of the head. Take a vertical section down the central panel at the back of the head (e). Hold it at 90° to the head and cut it to the length determined by the guideline (f). Take a further section below this one. The hair length may now be graduated to remove weight in the nape by angling the cut across the section, as required.

12 Move to the adjacent panel of hair and repeat the process, as before. Make sure the panels are connected, or long hairs will be left between adjacent panels.

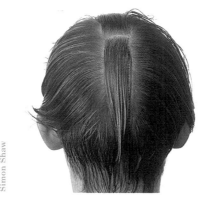

(e) Taking a vertical section at the back

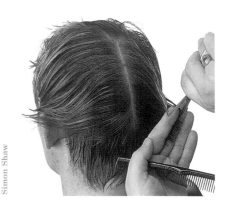

(f) Cutting to the required length

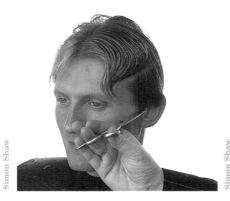

(g) Cutting the sides and sideburns

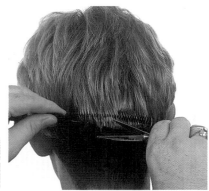

(h) Finishing the back

Tip

Remember to take into account that wet hair stretches, so do not cut it too short!

13 When the back is complete, move to one side of the head. If there are sideburns, note the required length and cut them to shape. Carefully outline the sideburn and the hair around the ears, then move down the sides of the nape with the tips of your scissors. Use the fingers of your other hand to guide and support the scissors or clippers whilst cutting (g).

14 Repeat this on the other side of the head. Ensure that the sideburns are level (see the tip on page 68). As you create the outlines, *make sure you do not cut into the natural hairline, particularly at the sides of the nape.*

15 Dry the hair into style.

16 Return to the centre panel of hair at the back of the head (h) and finish the nape area, the neckline and the side outlines, using scissors- or clippers-over-comb techniques.

17 Position the client's head so that it is bent forward slightly. Carefully cut the neckline straight across to the correct height (i). Use the proportions of the head and neck, the length of the hair and the position of the ears to determine the length that is most suitable. The neckline may be gently tapered to create a softer effect or the corners may be rounded, if required (j).

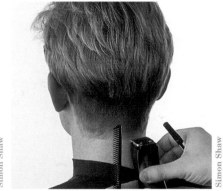
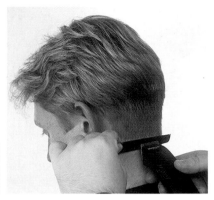

(i) **Cutting the neckline square**   (j) **Tapering the neckline**

18 Shave the areas outside the haircut outlines, if necessary (see Chapter 11).

19 Graduate the outlines to blend them with the skin, where required.

20 Finish the shape by combing, styling and dressing the hair into place (k).

(k) **The finished look**

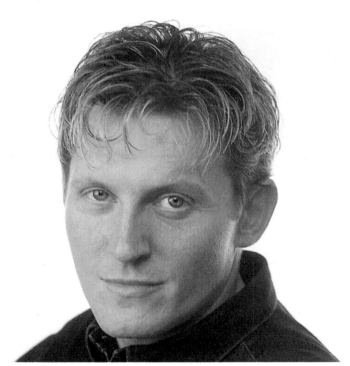

Tip

When cutting a squared neckline, the centre of the neckline should be cut slightly higher than at the sides to compensate for the skin in the centre of the neck moving further up as the head goes forward. The difference should be about 5mm. This will appear level when the head is returned to its normal position.

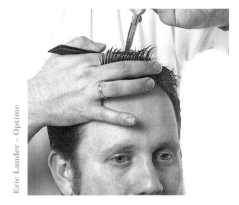

(a) Before cutting

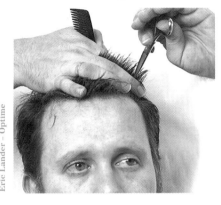

(b) Sectioning across the head

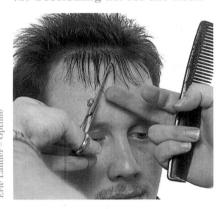

(c) Point cutting the front

Short graduation, tapered neckline, freehand cutting and scissor thinning

A tapered neckline (without a detachable comb clipper attachment).

1 Protect the client's clothes.

2 Comb the hair carefully, disentangling where required.

3 Wet the hair and move to the top of the head. Take a section of hair at the crown using the clubbing-over-fingers technique. Point cut into the ends of the hair section until the hair is at the required length. This will reduce the length and thin the hair to make it a less solid shape. Move across the head taking small sections and ensure that each panel of hair is connected, as before (a, b).

4 Using a freehand point cutting technique cut into the hair at the front to create differing lengths that will add definition and texture (c).

5 Roughly dry the hair (d).

6 Move to one side, or in the centre panel of hair at the back of the head, and begin cutting the hair using scissors- or clippers-over-comb techniques to the length of cut you require (e).

7 Move to the panel of hair adjacent to where you started and repeat the process, as before. Make sure you follow the cutting guideline from the previous section and adjacent panel (f).

8 Keep working around the head cutting the hair to the length determined by the chosen haircut shape.

9 As the shape develops keep looking in the mirror to make sure that it is symmetrical. Consult with your client at regular intervals to confirm that the developing shape is correct, making adjustments if required.

10 Note the required length for any sideburns that may be present, ensure they are level (see tip on page 68) and cut them to shape. Carefully outline the sideburn and around the ears then down the sides of the nape with the tips of your scissors or with the clippers (g).

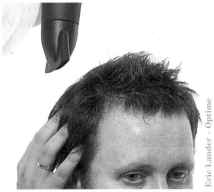

(d) Rough dry

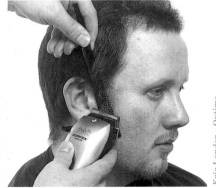

(e) Cut to required length

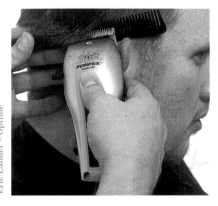

(f) Following the guidelines

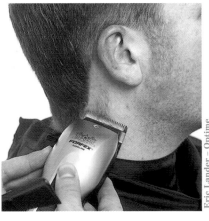

(g) Outlining the sideburns

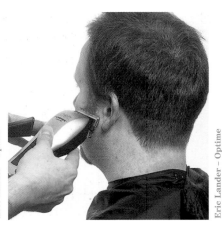

(h) Creating outlines

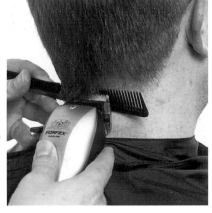

(i) Cutting the neckline

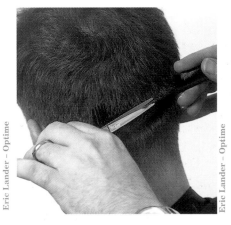

(j) The centre back panel

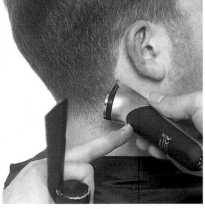

(k) Shaving outside the outlines

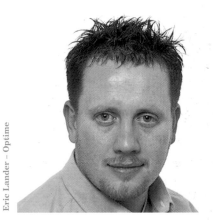

(l) The finished look

11 Repeat this on the other side of the head. *Make sure you do not cut into the natural hairline when creating the outlines, particularly at the sides of the nape* (g).

12 Position the client's head so that it is bent forward slightly and carefully cut the neckline to the correct height (i).

13 Move back to the centre panel of hair at the back of the head. Using either scissors- or clippers-over-comb techniques, begin to blend the hair where the top of the taper meets the hair on the top of the head. Move across the head taking small sections and ensure each panel is connected to blend the two areas together to create an even, continuous effect (j).

14 Shave the areas outside the haircut outlines, if required (see Chapter 11) or remove any visible hair using close cutting clippers (k).

15 Graduate the outlines to blend them with the skin, where required.

16 Finish the shape by combing, styling and dressing the hair into place (l).

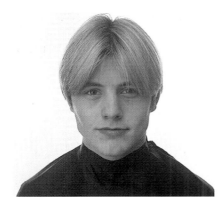

(a) Before cutting

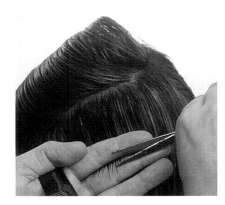

(b) Cutting the first section

Tip

When determining the correct height for the neckline you should consider the length of the neck, the position of the ears, the head shape and the length of the hair. If the neckline is too low on a short neck it will make the neck appear shorter; whilst if it is too short on a long neck it will make the neck appear longer. The best height is usually about 3–4cm below an imaginary line between the bottom of the ears, but always consider your client's wishes before cutting.

Graduated layers

In men's hairdressing, graduated layers are often required on the back and sides of the haircut to produce taller, leaner shapes that are more flattering to most men.

1 Protect the client's clothes (a).
2 Comb the hair carefully, disentangling it where required.
3 With the hair wet, make a parting about 2cm above the hairline, going from the front to the sides, around the ears and down into the nape.
4 Comb the hair at the front of the ear down from this parting to its natural position. Lift it by the width of two fingers to create the required amount of graduation. Cut the hair to the required length (b).
5 Take another section adjacent to the first, and cut it as before (c).
6 At the back of the ear, comb the hair forwards towards the ear, lift it the width of two fingers, and cut it to the guideline from the previous section.
7 Continue cutting the hair along this first section until you reach the nape.
8 Make the second parting above and parallel to the first. Start at the front and comb the hair to its natural fall, then lift it to the same position as before. Cut this section to the guideline created by the first section beneath.
9 Continue down the second parting, taking each section to exactly the same position where you held the hair from the first parting. Ensure that the hair is lifted by the same amount each time, or the graduation will not be consistent.
10 Make further partings, continuing up the head. Pull each section of hair to the same position and cut it to the same guideline.
11 Move to the other side and repeat the process. Ensure that the hair is pulled to the position equivalent to that on the previous side.

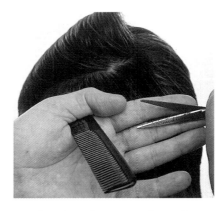

(c) Cutting the second section

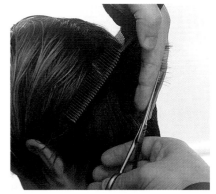

(d) Cross-checking the back

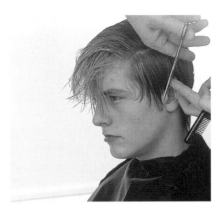

(e) Outlining

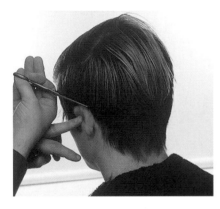

(f) Outlining

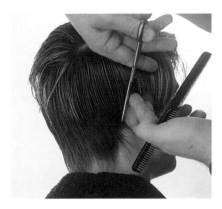

(g) Outlining

12 As the shape develops, keep looking in the mirror to make sure that the shape is symmetrical. Consult with your client at regular intervals to confirm that the developing shape is correct, making adjustments if required.

13 When both sides are complete, cross-check the back area to ensure that the shape is balanced and that the cut is accurate (d). This may be carried out with either scissors-over-fingers or scissors-over-comb techniques.

14 When the back is complete, move to one side of the head. If there are sideburns, note the required length and cut this sideburn to shape. Carefully outline the sideburn and the hair around the ears (e, f), then move down the sides of the nape with the tips of your scissors. Use the fingers of your other hand to guide and support the scissors or clippers whilst cutting (g).

15 Repeat this on the other side of the head. Ensure that the sideburns are level (see the tip on page 68). As you create the outlines, *make sure you do not cut into the natural hairline, particularly at the sides of the nape.*

16 Dry the hair into style.

17 Return to the centre panel of hair at the back of the head and finish the nape area, the neckline and the side outlines, using scissors- or clippers-over-comb techniques. The neckline should be squared, tapered or rounded, as required.

18 Shave the areas outside the haircut outlines, if necessary (see Chapter 11).

19 Graduate the outlines to blend them with the skin, where required.

20 Finish the shape by combing, styling and dressing the hair into place (h).

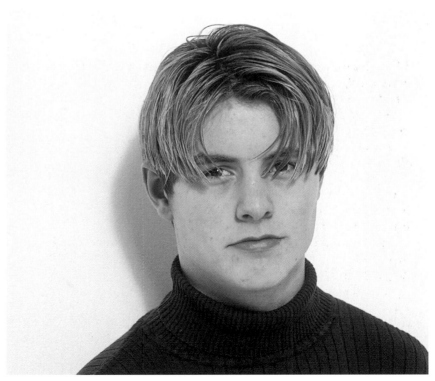

(h) The finished look

(h) Alternate finished look

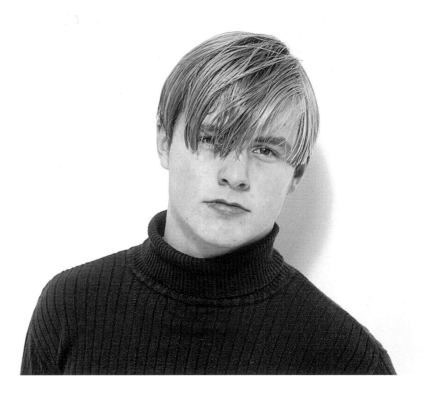

The sculpture cut, 'number 1' or skin fade

Different variations of the sculpture cut are popular with many men, but most often with young men. The name is derived from the closeness of the cut: it closely follows the features of the head, so the hair appears to be sculpted. It is also sometimes called a 'number 1' after the size of the clipper comb attachment often used to achieve the cut. Longer versions of this type of cut have been called 'number 3' or 'number 4', again after the size of comb attachment used.

Traditionally this type of cut was called a crew cut (the length usually being equivalent to that produced with a number 4 comb attachment). However, the crew cut was often achieved with just scissors-over-comb techniques, and it required great skill to ensure the same length of cut throughout.

The sculpture cut produces a very masculine shape. It can be quite severe, though variations in length may be used to produce effects to suit the individual client's requirements. The looks created are very easy to manage as no blow-styling or dressing is required. Some men who are partly bald enjoy these looks because the shortness of the hair reduces the effect and impact of the bald areas.

The sculpture cut is particularly suitable for very tight curly hair, where the hair is often taken very close. Indeed, the clippers are sometimes used at the back and sides with no comb attachment, and a skin fade is produced. Adjustable-blade clippers are usually set to their longest setting (equal to a size 1 blade), and the detachable clippers are used with a clipper blade of size 1 or above. Lines and shapes can be channelled (sometimes known as tramlining when used to create simple lines) into the hair on these styles to create elaborate designs.

Skin fade back and sides

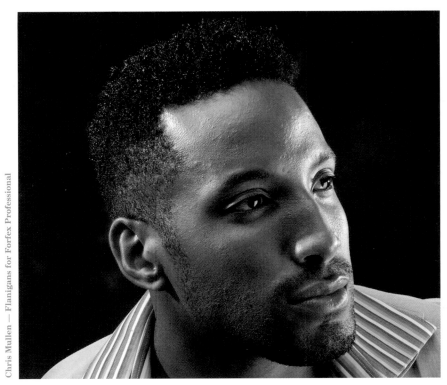

Chris Mullen — Flanigans for Forfex Professional

1 Protect the client's clothes.

2 Comb the hair carefully, disentangling it where required (a).

3 Start in the centre panel of hair at the back of the head. Begin cutting the hair using the clippers set to the longest setting or with a size 1 blade. Alternatively, a comb attachment can be used for a less severe effect. The best-sized comb for this look is either a number 1 or a number 2. Before you start, make sure that any comb attachment is securely attached to the clippers.

4 Place the clippers flat against the neck, just below the neckline. Using a *smooth, continuous movement*, push the clippers slowly up the head, keeping them flat against the scalp until you reach the area where you want the taper to begin: in this case the occipital bone. In a smooth *rocking* movement, *pivot* the clippers away from the head to produce the shape and length of hair that you want. Unless the top panels are to be cut this short as well,

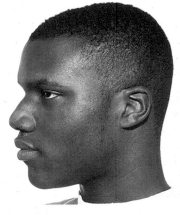

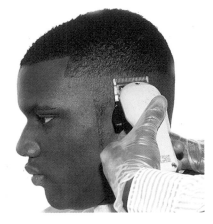

MK Hair Studio

(a) Before cutting

(b) Cutting the side

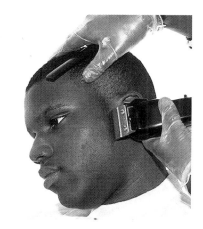

(c) Outlining around the ears

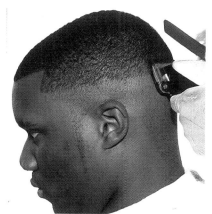

(d) Blending the back and top

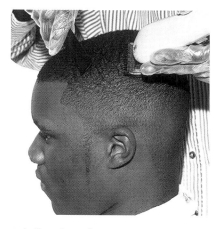

(e) Cutting the top

do not go higher than the occipital bone without pivoting away from the head.

5 Move to an adjacent panel of hair, and repeat the process as before. Make sure the panels are connected, or long hairs will be left between them.

6 Keep working around the head, cutting the hair to the length determined by the chosen haircut shape (b).

7 As the shape develops, keep looking in the mirror to make sure that the shape is even and symmetrical. Consult with your client at regular intervals to confirm that the developing shape is correct, making adjustments if required.

8 Move to one side of the head. If there are sideburns, note the required length for any sideburns and cut this sideburn to shape. Carefully outline the sideburn and the hair around the ears (c), then, having removed any comb attachment, move down the sides of the nape with the clippers. Use the fingers of your other hand to guide and support the clippers whilst cutting.

9 Repeat this on the other side of the head. Ensure that the sideburns are level (see the tip on page 68). As you create the outlines, *make sure you do not cut into the natural hairline*.

10 Position the client's head so that it is bent forward slightly. Carefully cut the neckline to the correct height. Use the proportions of the head and neck, the length of the hair and the position of the ears to determine the length that is most suitable.

11 The neckline must be tapered to create either a natural effect, or a skin fade effect where the hair appears to fade away. Do not cut it straight across. Use clippers-over-comb techniques and set the clippers to cut at the shortest setting, or use a size 000 blade. On longer hair, the bottom edge of the comb should be held against the skin and the clippers moved up or across the comb: the comb must be angled so that the hair will be cut shorter at the bottom and left longer towards the top. On very short hair the clippers are held directly against the scalp. Pivoting the clippers away in a smooth rocking movement blends and fades the neckline.

12 Return to the centre panel of hair at the back of the head. Using a number 1 comb attachment, or a size suitable for the length of hair required, begin to blend the hair where the top of the taper

Tip

Always comb the hair after each movement with the clippers, to remove loose hairs and ensure that you can see clearly.

Remove excess hair cuttings from the client's face and neck at regular intervals, to ensure that he is comfortable.

MK Hair Studio

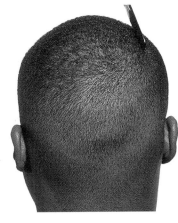

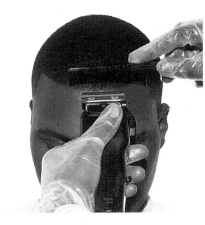

(f) An even result

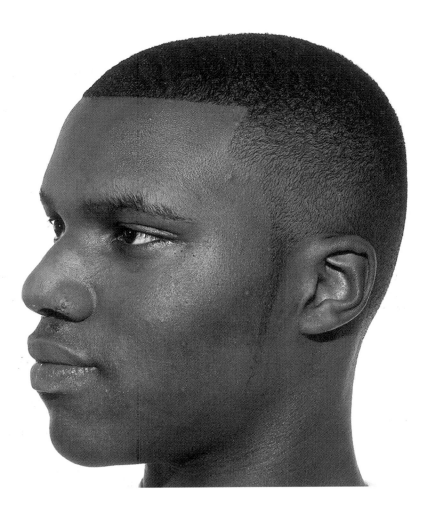

(g) Shaping the front hairline

(h) The finished look – skin fade back and sides and lined out front

meets the hair on the crown of the head (d). Move across the head, working on small sections and ensuring that each panel is connected to the previous one, blending the two areas together to create an even, continuous effect with no lines.

13 Move across the head, following the direction of hair growth. As you cut, ensure that successive panels of hair are connected (e).

14 Blend together the top panels and the side and back panels where they meet, to create an even, continuous effect (f). You may need to remove the comb attachment to do this.

15 The front hairline may be shaped with the clippers, if required, but avoid making deep cuts into the natural hairline (g).

16 Channelling with the clippers may now be used to create lines, shapes and designs, if required.

17 Comb all the hair through, checking for any long hairs. Remove them with scissors- or clippers-over-comb or freehand cutting techniques. If possible, rinse the hair first to remove the loose hairs and help make any longer hairs more visible.

18 Shave the areas outside the haircut outlines, if necessary (see Chapter 11).

19 Graduate the outlines to blend them with the skin, where required.

20 Finish the shape by combing the hair into place (h).

Longer layered looks

Uniform layers (including razor-thinning)

In men's hairdressing uniform layering is not often used throughout the whole haircut, because the shape produced is too round, though it can be used to create some suitable shapes on curly hair. Uniform layering is most often used through the top of the head, with graduated layering being used at the back and sides to produce a taller, leaner and more masculine shape.

1   Protect the client's clothes (a).
2   Comb the hair carefully, disentangling it where required.
3   With the hair wet, section the hair in two by making a parting from ear to ear across the top of the head. Take a section parallel to this parting at the crown, and hold it at 90° to the head. Cut it to length using the scissors-over-fingers technique. Make sure you cut the section straight across at 90° to the head (b).
4   Take a section going down the centre panel towards the front hairline (c). Hold this at 90° to the head and cut it to the same length. Continue down this panel, but do not cut the front section at this stage.
5   Take the front section forwards and hold it at 90° to the head. Cut it to the required length for the front (d). Remember that wet hair stretches, so do not cut it too short.
6   Return to the crown area and take a small section, again parallel to the first parting, and hold it at 90° to the head. Cut it to length following the guideline from the first section. Continue working forward down the centre panel, always cutting to the guideline from the previous section.
7   Move to the adjacent panel of hair and repeat the process. Make sure that the panels are connected.
8   Keep working around the top of the head, cutting the hair to the length determined by the chosen haircut shape.
9   Transfer the guideline down onto the side of the head by taking a vertical section (e). Continue cutting these sections to the required length. The hair length may be graduated to remove

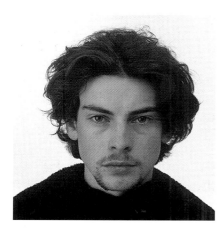

(a) Before cutting

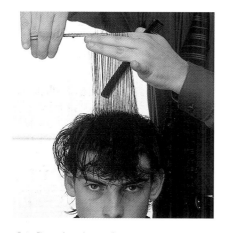

(b) Sectioning the crown

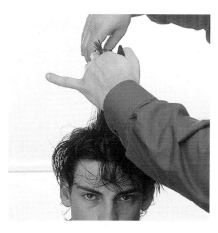

(c) Cutting the central panel

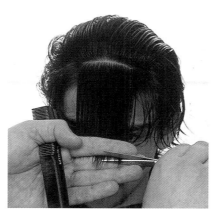

(d) Cutting the front section

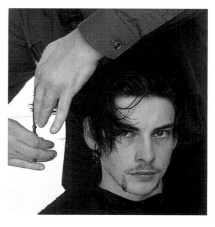

(e) Transferring the guideline to the sides

weight around the ears, by angling the cut across the section as required (f).

10   As the shape develops, keep looking in the mirror to make sure that the shape is symmetrical. Consult with your client at regular intervals to confirm that the developing shape is correct, making adjustments if required.

11   Transfer the guideline from the front of the first parting at the crown area through into the back of the head (g). Take a vertical section down the central panel at the back of the head. Hold it at 90° and cut it to the length determined by the guideline. Take a further section below this one. The hair length may now be graduated to remove weight in the nape, by angling the cut across the section as required.

12   Move to the adjacent panel of hair, and repeat the process as before. Make sure the panels are connected or long hairs will be left between them.

13   When the back is complete, move to one side of the head (h). If there are sideburns, note the required length and cut this sideburn to shape. Carefully outline the sideburn and the hair around the ears, then move down the sides of the nape with the tips of your scissors. Use the fingers of your other hand to guide and support the scissors or clippers whilst cutting.

14   Repeat this on the other side of the head. Ensure that the sideburns are level (see the tip on page 68). As you create the outlines, *make sure you do not cut into the natural hairline, particularly at the sides of the nape*.

15   Cut the neckline to the shape required by the look.

16   The top layers are then cut with a razor to reduce the thickness and to create more texture and movement. The hair must be wet, so dampen it again with a water spray, if necessary. Comb the hair straight back and start in the centre panel at the front, about 3cm back from the hairline. Do not start too near the hairline or the resulting short hairs will stick straight up! The hair is then cut, using gentle slicing movements with the razor. The razor and comb should move down the section together as the required amount of hair is removed (i, j). Take great care, as the razor can easily cut the hair straight through.

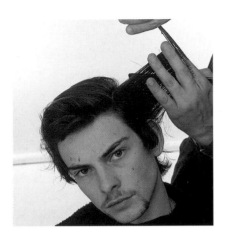

(f) Cutting the side

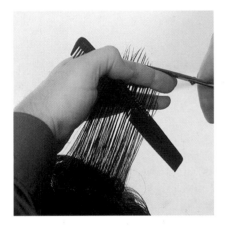

(g) Transferring the guideline to the back

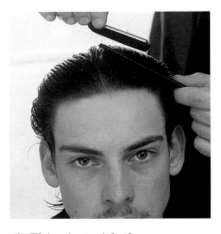

(i) Thinning with the razor

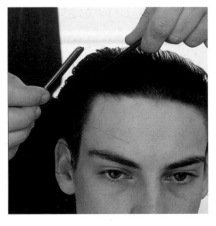

(j) Thinning with the razor

(h) Cutting the sides

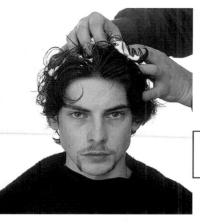

17   Shave the areas outside the haircut outlines, if necessary (see Chapter 11).

18   Graduate the outlines to blend them with the skin, where required.

19   Finish the shape by combing, styling and dressing the hair into place (k, l, m).

Tip

Make sure you cut each section on the top straight across at 90° to the head or a uniform layered effect will not be achieved.

(k) Applying finishing products

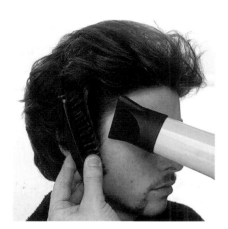

(l) Drying the hair

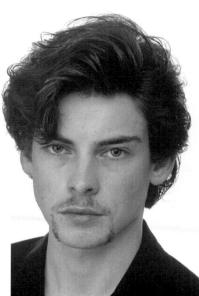

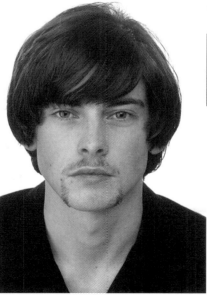

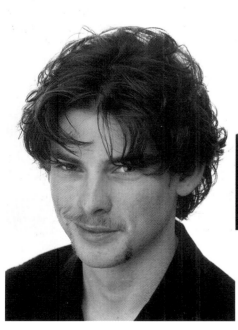

(m) Finished looks

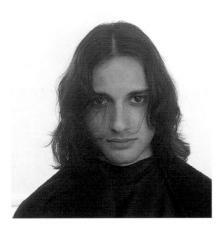

(a) Before cutting

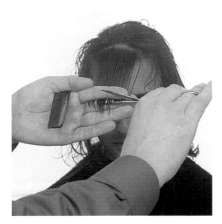

(b) Cutting the front

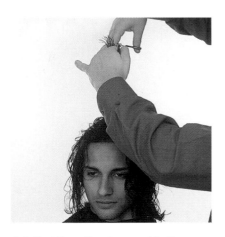

(c) Cutting the top guideline from the sides

Square layers

Square layers are good for creating movement and texture through the interior of a mid-length haircut. On men they are particularly suitable for longer haircuts because they produce a shape that is more square and angular, and thus more masculine. They also help make longer hair more manageable.

1 Protect the client's clothes (a).

2 Comb the hair carefully, disentangling it where required.

3 With the hair wet, make a centre parting from the forehead to the nape.

4 Create two sections in the nape, running slightly diagonally from the centre parting outwards to the bottom of the ears. Starting in the middle of these two sections, comb the hair down and cut it to the required length with the scissors-over-fingers technique. Continue cutting straight across these sections to produce a square line.

5 Take two more diagonal sections, about 2cm higher and running parallel to the first. Cut the hair to the guideline, sometimes called a baseline, which was created in the nape. Continue the baseline around onto the sides.

6 Continue working up the head, taking 2cm sections, until all of the hair at the back has been cut to this baseline.

7 Move to the front of the head and take a diagonal section about 2cm wide on the side from the centre parting to the top of the ears. Cut this section up from the baseline created at the bottom of the sides. Continue cutting up along the section to the required length for the hair at the front (b). Do not cut the front too short or the layers through the head will be too short.

8 Repeat this on the other side. Check that the sides are level.

9 Create a section going down the centre panel from the front hairline to the nape. Take the section at the front and hold the hair straight up at 90° to the head. Cut this to the guideline that will now be visible coming up from the sides (c). This will create a new guideline on the top that determines the length of the square layers throughout the interior of the haircut.

10 Continue cutting this guideline across the central panel to the crown area.

11 Take a next section of the central panel from below the crown area and comb it straight up to the same position as the last section on the top of the head. Cut this section to the guideline on the top to produce a square layer and retain the length at the back (d). Repeat this down the rest of the central panel, making sure that the hair is all combed straight up to the same position and cut to the top guideline.

12 Move to the adjacent panel of hair at the back and repeat the process, making sure that the panels are connected.

13 Keep working around the crown (e). Imagine that the crown is the hub of a wheel, and the panels of hair are each of the spokes. Follow this process until the hair at the back is connected with the hair at the sides.

Tip

Outlines can be achieved by cutting the hair with either close-cutting clippers or an electric razor. The outline hair may also be removed completely by shaving with a razor, which should be used following the shaving procedure described in Chapter 11, 'Shaving'.

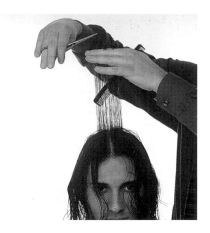

(d) Cutting a section from the back

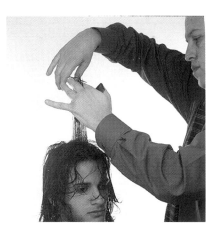

(e) Working round the crown

14 If there are sideburns, note the required length and cut them to shape. Ensure that they are level (see the tip on page 68).

15 Remove any unwanted hair from outside the outline, shaving these areas if necessary (see Chapter 11).

16 Finish the shape by combing, styling and dressing the hair into place (f).

(f) The finished look

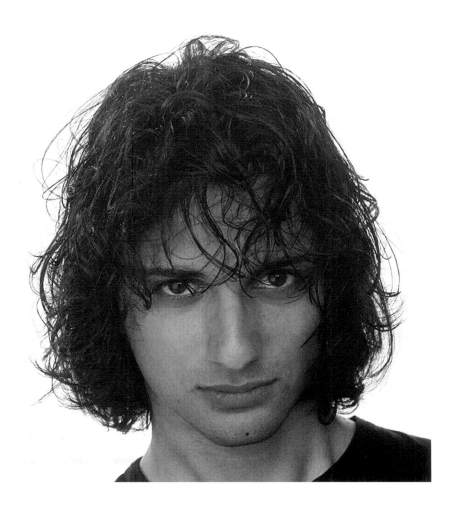

Finishing

When possible the hair should be rinsed after cutting to remove any loose hair cuttings, particularly on very short styles as the short hairs can be difficult to remove.

Styling products may then be applied, and the hair dried and dressed in accordance with the requirements of the desired look. Use the mirror regularly to check the balance and symmetry of the shape as you dress it.

Show the client the finished result and apply final finishing products if required. Provide advice and tips on after-care styling and products, as appropriate.

Health and safety

It is important to consider health and safety when cutting hair because of the risks associated with using electricity and the risk of cutting the skin. Here are some important health and safety factors that you must consider when providing haircutting services:

Avoid infection

- If the client has any cuts or abrasions on his head, or you suspect that an infection or infestation is present, you must not carry out the haircut.
- Pay special attention to hygiene when cutting hair, because of the risk of cross-infection through open cuts.
- Use only clean tools and equipment. Use alcoholic wipes and sprays to keep clippers clean and disinfected between clients.

Work safely with razors

- Open and safety razors have very sharp blades and must always be handled and used with great care.
- When it is not being used or when it is being carried, always close the handle to protect the blade of an open razor.
- Never place razors or other cutting tools in your pockets.
- Always sterilise a fixed-blade razor before *each* use.
- When using a detachable-blade open razor, always use a new blade for *each* new client.
- Used razor blades, called sharps, must be disposed of correctly in accordance with your salon policy. Soiled disposable materials should be placed in sealed plastic bags for removal.

Work safely with electricity

- Always handle and use electrical equipment with care, and in accordance with the manufacturers' instructions.

- Never place or use electric clippers or other electrical equipment near water.
- Do not go near electrical equipment that is lying in water – first switch off the power at the mains.
- Before commencing work, visually check that electrical equipment is safe to use. Check that the cable has not frayed or been pulled, and that the plug is not loose.
- When using and storing electrical equipment, pay attention to the position of cables.
- Never overload sockets. Do not plug too many items of electrical equipment into the same socket.
- Follow the manufacturers' instructions for the care of your scissors and clippers. To avoid damage, be sure to clean and lubricate the blades regularly.
- Electrical equipment must be regularly tested, and given a certificate of testing confirming that it is safe for use. The salon owner will ensure that this is carried out, as required.

Be prepared for accidents

- Make sure that you know the whereabouts of your salon's first-aid kit.
- Keep yourself up to date with your salon's first-aid and accident procedures.
- If the client's skin is cut while you are cutting his hair, stay calm and explain what has happened. Follow your salon's first-aid and accident procedures.

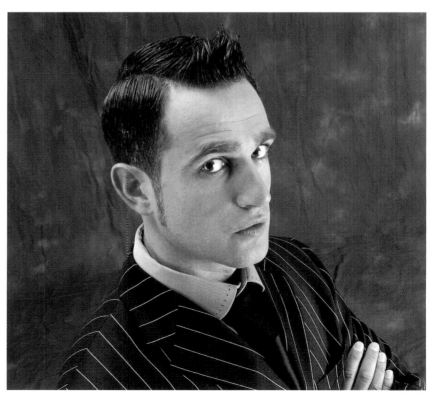

Chris Mullen – Flanigans for Forfex Professional

Here is an example of what you should do. Give the client a clean dressing and ask him to apply it against the cut until the bleeding stops. A new dressing or plaster may then be applied. **Do not touch the cut yourself.** If the cut is more serious, advise the client to seek medical attention as soon as possible. If any gowns or towels have been soiled, seal them in a plastic bag and launder them at a high temperature as soon as possible.

- If you cut your *own* skin while you are cutting a client's hair, stay calm and explain what has happened. Follow your salon's first-aid and accident procedures.

Here is an example of what you should do. Excuse yourself from the client and rinse the cut under cold running water to remove any hairs. Apply a clean dressing against the cut, until the bleeding stops. A new dressing or plaster may then be applied. If the cut is more serious, seek medical attention as soon as possible. If any gowns or towels have been soiled, seal them in a plastic bag and launder them at a high temperature as soon as possible.

Activities

1   Research the options available for reconditioning scissors. Produce a report setting out the features and benefits of each option and present this to your manager. With the manager's permission, recommend the best options to your colleagues.

2   Visit local wholesalers and use the Internet to search manufacturers' sites to research the types of electric clippers and trimmers and blades and attachments that are available. Produce a chart showing the features and benefits of each item, especially noting things like ease of use, maintenance requirements, life expectancy and any unique features. You can then use the information to help you and your colleagues choose the equipment that is most suitable for your requirements.

Check your knowledge

1   Describe the main purpose of cutting hair.

2   Describe why outlines are important in men's haircutting.

3   Explain why most men wear sideburns.

4   Describe the three main neckline shapes in men's hairdressing.

5   Outline the best way of dealing with a double crown.

6   Describe the condition thought to be the cause of male-pattern alopecia.

7   Describe the looks usually most suitable for men with male-pattern alopecia.

8   Describe how added hairpieces are secured to the head.

9 Describe the look least suited to a client with a round face.

10 State the cutting length of a size 1 clipper blade.

11 Why must clipper blades be checked before use and especially after being dismantled?

12 Describe how to identify a client's natural parting.

13 State which cutting technique(s) should be carried out on dry hair and not carried out on wet hair.

14 Describe the angle of graduation produced if you hold a section of hair at 90° to the head and club cut it at 90°.

15 State why it is important to establish and follow the correct cutting guideline.

16 Describe how to make sure that sideburns are cut level.

17 Describe the action that should be taken if, about to cut a client's hair, you suspect an infestation is present on their head.

18 Describe the action you should take if you were to cut yourself whilst cutting a client's hair.

Drying and finishing men's hair

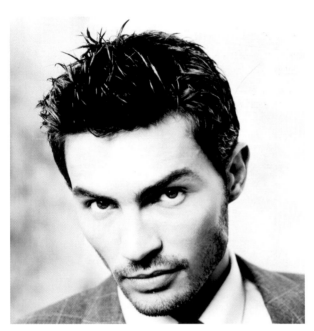

6

Goldwell

Learning objectives

Blow-drying is the art of styling wet hair with brushes, combs or fingers whilst blow-drying it with a hand-held hairdryer. Today, many men enjoy having their hair shampooed and 'blow-styled', so the barber must consider how the hair is to be professionally dried and finished.

The techniques used for blow-drying and styling men's hair are very similar to those used in women's hairdressing. Some would say there is no difference, but the barber understands that differences exist in the way that the techniques are used, and in the different effects that they achieve.

This chapter examines how blow-drying and styling techniques are used in men's hairdressing. It covers the following topics:

- **the theory of blow-drying**
- **consultation for blow-drying**
- **preparation for blow-drying**
- **styling products, tools and equipment**
- **blow-drying techniques – including blow-waving, finger drying, scrunch drying and natural drying**
- **finishing techniques**
- **health and safety**

The theory of blow-drying

Blow-drying works by temporarily changing the hair structure.

Wet hair is very elastic and can stretch by up to 50 per cent of its original length. It is stretchy because the weaker hydrogen bonds and salt links, which form part of the hair cortex (see page 17), are temporarily broken. The application of heat then softens the hair and causes it to stretch and mould to the new shape created by the brush, comb or fingers. The hair structure has now changed from its original state, called the alpha state (not stretched) to the beta state (stretched).

The new shape is only temporary because hair is hygroscopic: it absorbs moisture. Eventually moisture from the atmosphere will enter the hair and it will return to its natural alpha state. Washing the hair in hot water will return the hair to its natural state immediately.

Consultation prior to blow-drying

Blow-drying is usually carried out following a shampoo or haircut, where it is used to produce the final look that the haircut has created. Consultation for blow-drying is likely to have been included in the consultation *before* the haircut, but you must still make sure that time is always set aside to discuss the client's requirements with him.

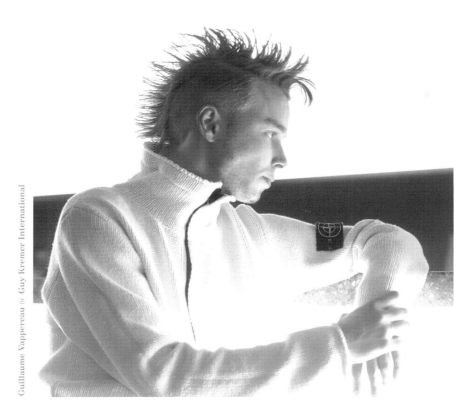

Guillaume Vappereau @ Guy Kremer International

Here are some of the factors that must be considered when blow-drying men's hair.

- Identify the client's requirements. Give him advice on suitable styles and agree the final effect to be achieved.
- Look for signs of any unusual hair growth patterns.
- Identify the natural fall of the hair.
- Determine whether the hair is coarse or fine.

Many men prefer not to have too much volume created in the finished blow-dried style. You should pay particular attention to this during the consultation and ensure that you choose suitable brushes and techniques for creating the amount of volume required.

It may also be helpful if you read Chapter 2, 'Client care for men'.

Preparation for blow-drying

Following the consultation and before you begin work, gather together all the products, tools and equipment you will require. You must also prepare the client and his hair.

Preparing the client

Remove any wet towels and make sure your client is comfortable. If the hair has just been cut, ensure that all the hair cuttings are removed.

Preparing the hair

1 Shampoo and towel-dry the hair.
2 Comb out any tangles using a comb with widely spaced teeth.
3 Apply a suitable blow-styling aid, if the hair or the style requires it. Tell your client why you advise using the styling aid and make sure your client agrees before you apply it!

Products, tools and equipment

Styling and finishing products

Recently, there has been a large increase in the range of styling and finishing products available that have been produced specifically for men. These products are designed to work well on different hair types and to support a wide range of style effects. They perform particularly well on short styles, which are worn by many men.

Men's products often contain little or no perfume and are available in packaging specifically designed to be attractive to men. These products work just as well on women's hair and can support many women's styles. Similarly, general styling products can be used equally well on men's hair.

Styling products are often versatile and many can be applied to the hair either before or after blow-drying, but some products are designed for use specifically before or after blow-drying. Products that are applied *before* are designed to protect the hair and help the styling process by providing added support to the style. Products that are applied *after* blow-drying impart shine and help to achieve and retain the finished style.

Some products bond to the internal structure of the hair and help the hair to retain moisture, as well as to retain the style. Yet others are designed to help the process of moulding and shaping the hair. A good knowledge of products and their use will help you to choose the most suitable products for creating different styles and effects.

Whatever they are intended to do, most styling products will contain one or more of the following.

- **Plasticisers** These coat the hair, help mould it to shape, and then support the finished hairstyle.
- **Moisturisers** These retain the hair's natural moisture while resisting the absorption of further moisture from the atmosphere.
- **Protectors** These protect the hair from the heat of the dryer and the adverse effects of the environment, particularly from the effects of ultra-violet rays from the sun.

Two types of products are especially common in men's hairdressing today.

- **Blow-styling aids** These are used to help mould the hair into shape. They support the finished hairstyle and protect the hair from the heat of the drying process, whilst also adding volume. They are available in a variety of strengths, ranging from 'firm hold' to 'ultra hold', and they are usually available as lotions, sprays, mousses and gels.

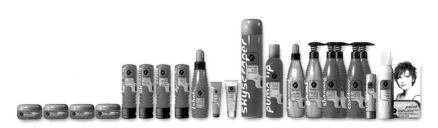

Fudge

- **Dressing and finishing aids** These are used to retain the finished style. Some aids can also increase the shine, and improve the apparent condition of the hair. They are often used to give definition and texture to selected sections of hair, particularly on short styles, and are commonly available as mousses, gels, creams, oils and waxes.

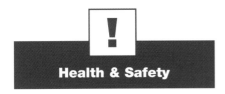

Health & Safety

Always observe high standards of hygiene in your work. Keep all brushes and combs clean. Make sure you wash them if they are dropped on the floor.

Tools

Brushes

Brushes are available in many different shapes and sizes. Next to the hairdryer they are probably the most important item you will need.

Each brush is designed for a particular purpose, although often, with experience, it is possible to achieve similar effects with different brushes. Some brushes are designed to help you dry the hair quickly and are good for general shaping. Others are good for creating volume or for creating waves.

Here are some brushes commonly used in men's hairdressing:

- **Half-round plastic brushes** These are good for creating smooth finishes and for general shaping (a). They can be used to build volume into the style during drying and can also be used to produce larger waves during blow-waving.
- **Half-round or straight bristle brushes** These can be either wood or plastic but in both cases they have short stiff bristles that grip the hair well (b, c). Bristle brushes are many barbers' preferred choice for blow-drying and especially blow-waving, as they can be used to produce large or small waves. They are often used to define partings and to control areas of hair without building too much volume into the style.
- **Vent brushes** Vent brushes (d) have vents which allow the air to flow through easily and so aid quick drying. They are very easy to use and are often used by barbers after drying, to break up the style and create a textured effect.

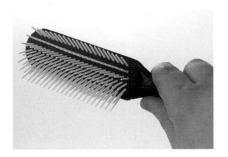

(a) Half-round plastic brush

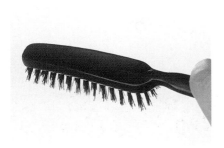

(b) Plastic bristle brush

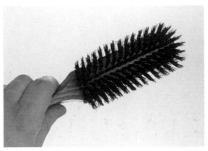

(c) Wooden bristle brush

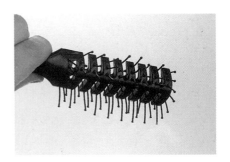

(d) Vent brush

- **Circular brushes** These are available in many different sizes. Small-diameter brushes are better for short to medium-length hair and produce a curled effect. Larger-diameter brushes work well on medium to long hair and produce a softer curl. Circular brushes are used more often for creating women's hairstyles than men's, but some may be used for blow-waving or for dealing with longer hair (e).

(e) Circular brush

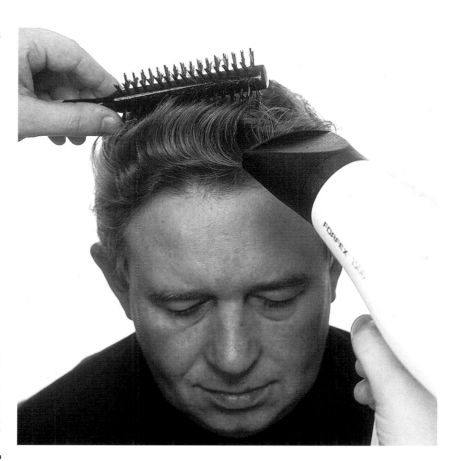

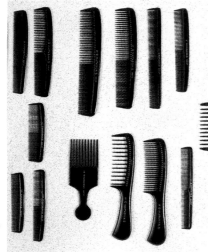

Combs

Combs required include wide-toothed combs for disentangling the hair after it has been shampooed, and cutting combs or straight combs for sectioning longer hair before blow-drying. Cutting combs may also be used for creating waves during blow-waving but they must be heat-resistant.

Metal combs too are available, and are used during blow-waving. They should be used with great care, as the metal can become quite hot from the heat of the dryer. Only professional combs should be used.

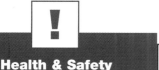

Health & Safety

Metal combs retain heat and can burn the scalp so take extra care when using them.

Tip

Always use a comb with widely spaced teeth for disentangling the hair, or the hair will pull and may break!

Equipment

The most important piece of blow-drying equipment is, of course, the hand-held hairdryer. There are many models to choose from, but essentially the dryer should have adjustable speeds and temperatures, and be light and easy to hold. A professional-quality dryer should be your preferred choice, as this will have several functions and be adequately constructed to give many years of trouble-free service with minimum maintenance.

The dryer must include a nozzle to concentrate and direct the airflow, which is particularly important for blow-waving and for men's hairdressing in general. The dryer should also have a diffuser, which disperses the airflow to dry the hair without moving it out of place. This method of drying produces an effect similar to that of natural drying and is often used in 'scrunch drying' (described below).

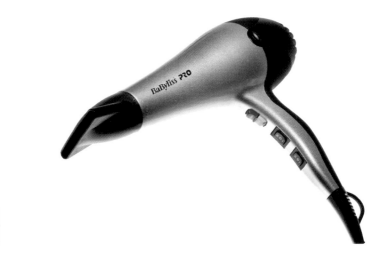

BaByliss

Blow-drying techniques

Your choice of blow-drying techniques will be based upon a number of important factors:

- the hair texture
- the natural hair fall
- the density (or quantity) of the hair
- the haircut
- the desired style.

Different types of hair may require different techniques and can produce different effects. Thick, coarse hair is often the easiest to blow-dry, as it can be moulded to produce strong effects; however, it can take longer to dry. Fine hair often requires the use of styling aids to help thicken the hair and support the finished style.

A variety of different blow-drying techniques may be used to create the different effects required in men's hairdressing. Many of these techniques are also used to dry and style women's hair, but here we will consider their use for creating men's hairstyles.

Blow-drying

Blow-drying is drying the hair with a hand-held hairdryer. It can be used just to dry the hair, but it is usually used to dry the hair into a shape or style.

A blow-drying method

1 Towel-dry the hair and apply styling aids, as required (a).

2 Disentangle the hair, using a comb with widely spaced teeth.

3 If the hair is long, cleanly divide it into small sections, using plain clips if required. If the hair is short, use the brush to divide the area of hair you are going to dry into manageable sections. Take horizontal sections for hair that is to go down, and vertical sections for hair that is to go back.

4 Lift the section of hair with the brush, and direct the heated airflow at the root area first – but not at the scalp, or it will burn. The angle at which you lift the hair will determine the amount of volume that is created (b).

5 Work methodically and ensure that you keep any wet hair away from the hair you are drying, or have already dried. Use plain clips to secure the hair, if required. (Remember: try not to use brightly coloured clips as these might embarrass your client!)

6 During drying, always direct the airflow *away* from the roots and *towards* the ends of the hair (c). Do not direct the airflow from the ends to the roots, or the cuticles will be blown open and the hair will become dull, rough and easily tangled.

7 Keep moving the brush as you direct the warm air over the section you are drying. Visualise the moulding process that is taking place as you manipulate the dryer, brush and hair (d). Make sure the section is fully dry. If the hair is long, allow it to cool before removing your brush – or use the cold-air button on your dryer if it has one.

8 Finish the style by dressing with combs or brushes. Apply finishing products, if required.

Tip

Many men prefer not to have too much volume created in the finished blow-dried style. Make sure you use the correct angle of lift to achieve the amount of volume required.

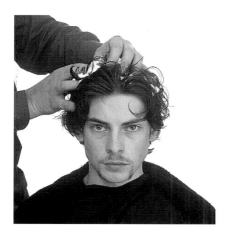

(a) Apply styling aids

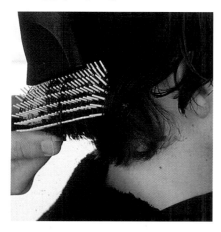

(b) Lift the hair with a brush

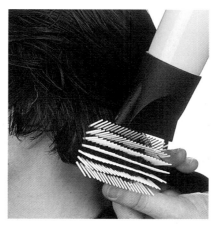

(c) Direct the airflow

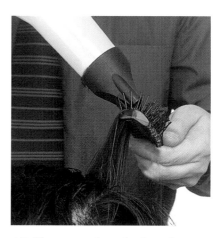

(d) Keep moving the brush

Tip

When blow-drying, use the mirror regularly to check the balance of the style as it develops.

Health & Safety

Check that the temperature setting on your dryer is correct prior to starting work. Test that the temperature is suitable by directing the airflow against the back of your hand.

Take care not to burn the hair or scalp by leaving the airflow directed in one place for too long.

Blow-waving

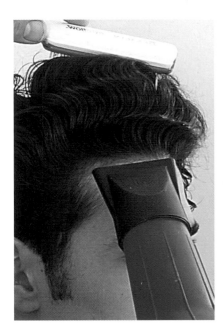

Vidal Sassoon

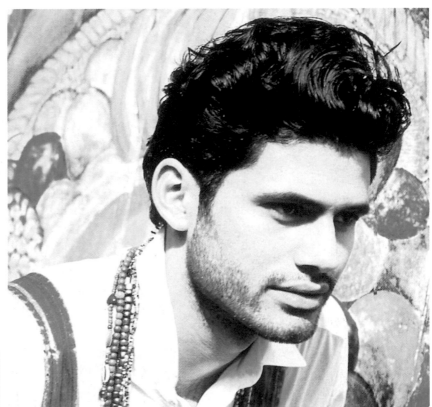

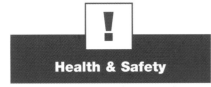

Health & Safety

Take extra care not to burn the scalp when blow-waving, as the nozzle also concentrates the heat!

At one time blow-waving was very popular in men's hairdressing. Many men would have waves styled into their hair. Some had them going straight back; others had them going forward; yet others used waves in partings or at the sides to control the hair and keep it brushed back. Today, blow-waving is sometimes seen as being old-fashioned, and people visualise a head full of tightly formed waves. Indeed, styles full of very visible waves are not currently in vogue, but the barber understands that blow-waving skills are essential in men's hairdressing.

Tip

Blow-waving is much easier to achieve if you use a nozzle on the dryer.

Always towel-dry the hair before blow-waving, but make sure that the hair is still quite damp or the waves will not form.

Tip

Do not keep trying to create waves on dry hair – use a water spray and start again!

Tip

Blow-waving is a skill that takes a lot of practice to develop. Good co-ordination is required in both hands. Practise by blow-waving just three consecutive waves before you try to do more.

Blow-waving may only be used on hair that is over about 6cm in length, as the length of hair must be sufficient to allow the wave to form. It can be used very effectively to control unruly hair, particularly naturally curly or wavy hair. The waves should be created following the natural fall of the hair: this makes it easier to blow-wave and will ensure that the style is retained for as long as possible. It will also be much easier for clients to manage their own hair in this way.

Waves are often used *within* blow-drying to create movement that controls the hair and supports the style, in the same way that the hair may be permed to help support a desired style. The blow-drying is then completed with a vent brush, which breaks up the hair and leaves a casual finish with few or no waves visible.

A blow-waving method

1   Towel-dry the hair and apply styling aids as required. The hair should be left quite damp.

2   Disentangle the hair, using a comb with widely spaced teeth.

3   Start at the front hairline and follow the hair's natural movements.

4   With a suitable brush or a wide-toothed comb, make a backward movement for about 5cm and grip the hair. Turn the brush or comb slightly and, whilst gripping the hair, make a slight forward movement that produces the shape of a wave.

5   Direct the warm airflow along the trough created against the brush or comb, moving in the opposite direction to the brush or comb. Use a nozzle attachment on the dryer to concentrate the airflow (a).

6   Keep moving the airflow along the hair until the hair is dry, taking care not to burn the hair or scalp. Leave the hair to cool for a few seconds, or use the cold-air button on your dryer to fix the wave before moving on to the second wave.

7   The second wave is created in a similar way to the first, but in the opposite direction (b).

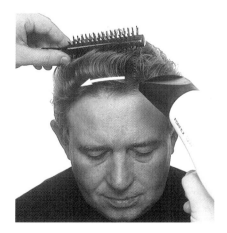
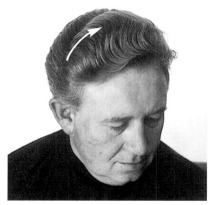

(a) Direct the airflow   (b) Create the second wave

8 Keep working through the hair, creating waves where required, following the hair's natural fall. Create each wave in the opposite direction to the previous one, until the style is complete.

9 The shorter areas of hair should be dried smoothly to follow the movement of the last wave and to meet the style requirements.

10 Finish the style by dressing with a comb, or use a vent brush for a broken or textured effect (c). Apply finishing products, if required (d).

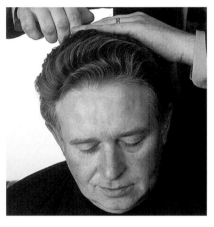

(c) Finish with a comb or brush

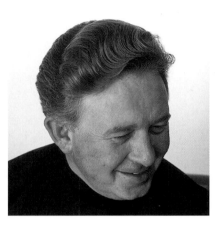

(d) The finished look

Contemporary blow-waving

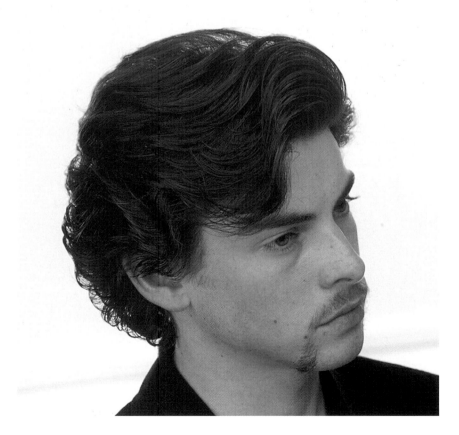

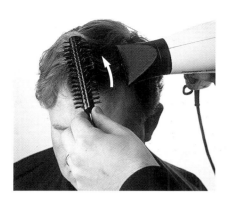

(a) First wave

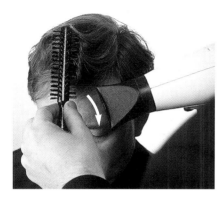

(b) Second wave

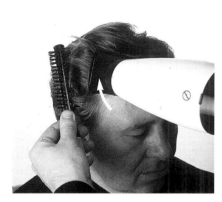

(c) Third wave

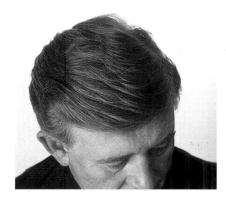

(d) The finished look

Blow-waving in contemporary styles

Blow-waving may be used to create movement that supports a wide range of styles. Many of these styles incorporate just three wave movements to achieve the required control and support.

The following method illustrates how blow-waving three consecutive wave movements may be used to produce a traditional style with a parting, without creating unwanted volume. This technique may then be applied in creating many different styles and effects.

1 Towel-dry the hair and apply styling aids as required. The hair should be left quite damp.

2 Disentangle the hair, using a comb with widely spaced teeth.

3 To find the natural parting, comb the hair back, then push it forward slightly with the palm of your hand. The hair will fall between the front hairline and the crown: this is the natural parting.

4 Start at the front hairline section of the parting.

5 With a suitable brush or wide-toothed comb, make a backward movement away from the parting for about 5cm and grip the hair. Turn the brush or comb slightly and, whilst gripping the hair, make a slight forward movement towards the parting, to produce the shape of a wave with the trough going up towards the crown.

6 Direct the warm airflow along the trough created against the brush or comb, moving in the opposite direction to the brush or comb (a).

7 Keep moving the airflow along the hair until it is dry, taking care not to burn the hair or scalp. Do not direct the airflow too deeply into the trough. The intention is to create movement, as opposed to a full wave. Let the hair rest for a few seconds or use your cold-air button to cool the hair and fix the movement before moving on to the second wave movement.

8 The second wave movement is created in a similar way to the first, but in the opposite direction. The movement is really a series of short movements with the dryer to mould the hair around the front hairline. The trough of the wave moves towards the face. Keep working through the hair until you reach the other side (b).

9 Make the third wave movement in the opposite direction, so that the trough of the wave goes back up towards the crown (c). You will notice that this turns the hair to go down or slightly back on the side opposite the parting.

10 The shorter areas of hair should be dried smoothly to meet the style requirements.

11 Finish the style by dressing with a comb, or use a vent brush for a more broken or textured effect. Apply finishing products, if required (d).

Other techniques

Finger drying

In finger drying the hair is styled by pulling, teasing and lifting with the fingers while the airflow from the dryer is used to mould the hair to the shape that has been created. The method results in fullness and soft billowing shapes which have little definition and so create a casual finished look.

Finger-dried looks

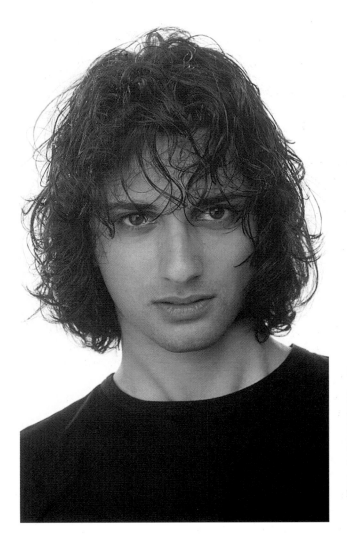

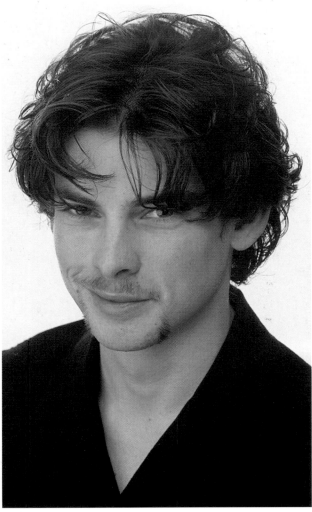

Scrunch drying

Scrunch drying is used more often in women's hairdressing than men's, primarily because it is usually used on longer hair to produce a casual, ruffled effect that is particularly suitable for women. It may be used on men, but a more masculine result is often required. Scrunch drying is usually carried out with a diffuser attachment on the dryer.

Scrunch drying

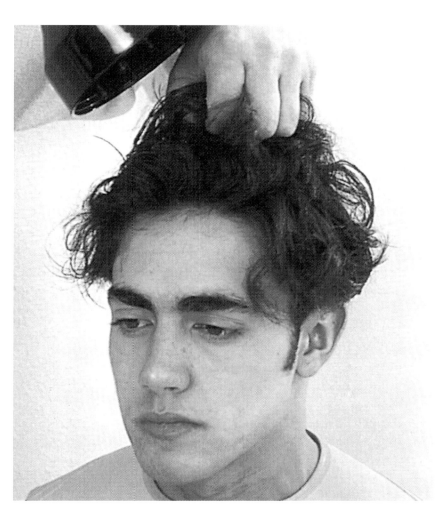

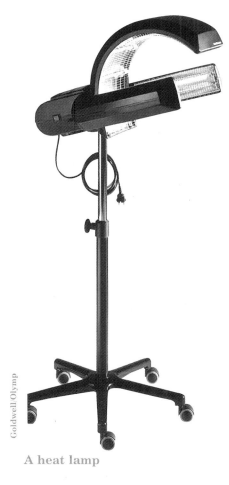

Goldwell Olymp

A heat lamp

Natural drying

Natural drying is simply leaving the hair to dry naturally. Some men choose natural drying when it suits the hairstyle they are wearing.

In the salon, natural drying is usually assisted by the application of heat from infrared lamps or accelerators or by blow-drying with a diffuser attachment. Essentially, the main characteristic of this method is that the hair is not styled during drying but is left to dry in its natural fall.

Finishing techniques

After drying, the style should be finished by combing or brushing. Some styling aids may be applied at this time to help smooth the hair while it is being dressed. Use of the comb will produce a smooth result, whereas a brush is likely to produce a more broken or textured effect. Use the mirror regularly to check the balance and symmetry of the style as you dress it.

When the desired effect has been achieved, finishing aids such as hairspray or wax may be applied to help retain it.

Health and safety

Everyone in the salon has a duty to work safely and keep his or her environment safe. It is important to consider health and safety in blow-drying, because of the risks associated with using electricity and the risk of burning the skin with the heat from the drying equipment.

Here are some important health and safety factors that you must consider when providing blow-drying services.

Work safely with electricity

- Electrical equipment must always be handled and used with care, in accordance with the manufacturers' instructions.
- Never use or place a hand-dryer or other electrical equipment near water.
- Do not go near electrical equipment that is lying in water – switch off the mains power first.
- Before commencing work, visually check that electrical equipment is safe to use – check that the cable has not frayed or been pulled, and that the plug is not loose.
- Pay attention to the position of cables when using and storing electrical equipment.
- Never overload sockets by plugging too many items of electrical equipment into the same socket.
- Electrical equipment must be regularly tested and given a certificate of testing to confirm that it is safe to use. Your salon owner will ensure that this is carried out, as required.

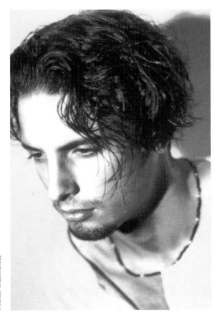

Vidal Sassoon

Avoid accidents

- Follow the manufacturer's instructions for the care of your dryer. Ensure that you clean the air filter regularly, to avoid overheating.
- Take care not to let the client's or your own hair or clothes get drawn into the air inlet at the back of the dryer.
- Always direct the airflow away from the scalp – this avoids burning, and produces a better, smoother blow-dried result.
- Use only clean tools and equipment.

Be prepared for accidents

- Make sure that you know the whereabouts of your salon's first-aid kit.
- Keep yourself up to date with your salon's first-aid and accident procedures.

Activities

1 Visit local wholesalers and research the styling and finishing products available for men's hairdressing. Organise your findings into product groups, based on what they do. Compare the different alternatives and shortlist those that provide the best features for your purposes. Compare this shortlist with the products in your salon. You can then recommend additional products to your manager.

2 Practise the blow-waving technique until you can link at least three consecutive waves together in a fluid, unbroken sequence before moving on to waving a full head.

Check your knowledge

1 Describe the changes that take place in the hair structure during blow-drying.

2 Describe the effect that a humid atmosphere has on blow-dried hair.

3 Describe the importance of considering volume when blow-drying men's hair.

4 List two things that should be done to prepare the client's hair before blow-drying.

5 State the purpose of plasticisers in a styling product.

6 What type of brush is most suitable for blow-waving?

7 What type of comb should be used for disentangling hair?

8 When should a nozzle should be used on a hand-held hairdryer?

9 Describe why it is important to consider air flow when blow-drying and blow-waving hair.

10 What should you do if the hair becomes dry before the style has been achieved?

11 Describe natural drying.

12 How do you check that hairdryers are safe to use?

13 What action should be taken if a hairdryer was accidentally left on a wet surface?

14 Why is it important to take care with the inlet of a hairdryer?

Colouring men's hair

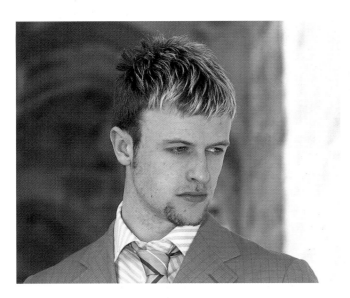

7

Guillaume Vappereau @ Guy Kremer International

Learning objectives

Traditionally, hair colouring has not often been required as a service in the barber's shop, so few barbers have developed or offered colouring services. Colouring has featured in some fashionable men's looks, such as the 'highlighted' looks that were popular in the 1980s. Partial hair colouring and lightening have been more popular with men: although some men have had full-head colours, usually to mask grey hairs, it has mostly been women who have requested colouring services. Today, it is still the case that few men have their hair coloured, but some have recognised that colouring can provide depth, tone and texture to enhance a new haircut or to make an old hairstyle more interesting.

This chapter is designed to provide an insight into how hair colouring, including bleaching, can be used in men's hairdressing. If you are new to colouring and bleaching and intend to become expert, you will need to undertake more detailed studies of the principles and techniques of colouring, which are mostly the same for both men and women. Detailed technical information on colouring and bleaching can be found in other books within the HABIA/Thomson Learning series.

Here are some of the topics covered in this chapter:

- **the basic principles of colouring**
- **the different types of hair colourants**
- **bleaching**
- **consultation for colouring men's hair**
- **colouring in men's hairdressing**

The basic principles of colouring

Before reading this section it may be helpful if you read Chapter 2, 'Client care for men'.

Some basic facts about colour

Colour helps us to interpret the world we see around us. Indeed, it is often used to provide information and instructions. Colour makes things appear more interesting and attractive. It can affect our moods, make things appear warm or cold, subdued or vibrant. On hair it can make subtle or dramatic changes to a person's appearance, benefits that have been recognised in hairdressing for many years.

Why we see colour

White light such as normal daylight is actually a mixture of light of many different colours. These become visible only when a prism scatters the light, or when raindrops scatter sunlight to display the different colours in a rainbow. The range of colours that we see, from red to violet, is called the visible spectrum.

The colours that we see are the result of different parts of the light being absorbed and reflected. Consider a red object, for example. When white light falls on this, the *red* light in the spectrum is *reflected*, and all of the *other* colours in the white light are *absorbed*. The reflected light is what reaches our eyes, so the object looks red.

Natural hair colour

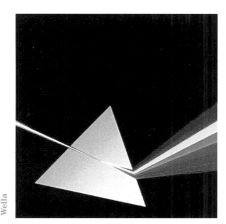

The colour spectrum from visible light

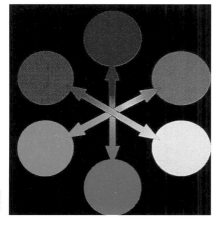

The colour circle

Melanin granules in the cortex of the hair (1μm is 1/1000th of 1mm)

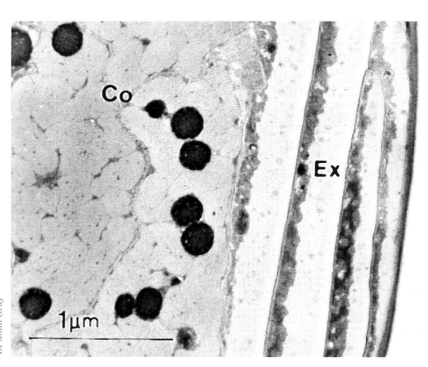

Tip

The hair colour we see is reflected light: a portion only of the light falling on the hair. Natural daylight contains the complete spectrum – all the colours of the rainbow. Artificial lights, however, contain only some of them. Fluorescent lights tend to neutralise red and warm colours, while tungsten lights tend to add warmth and reduce ash effects. Natural daylight is the best light for showing the true hair colour.

Colour pigments

The natural colour of hair is due to granules of a pigment called melanin. The type of this pigment, and how much there is of it, determines the colour.

Melanin is present within the hair cortex. The light falling on the hair passes through the hair cuticle, as this is translucent. The light is then reflected by the melanin. The colour we see is therefore determined by the colour that the melanin reflects.

There are two main types of melanin present in the hair:

- **Eumelanin** is responsible for black and brown hair
- **Pheomelanin** is responsible for red and blonde hair

Most people have a mixture of the two types of melanin in their hair. Their natural hair colour is formed by the quantity of each type of pigment that is present.

Going grey

Age and other factors such as stress can affect the production of natural hair pigments. As we get older, our new hairs have reduced levels of pigment – or, in the case of white hair, no pigment at all.

Over time, the proportion of hairs on the head with reduced pigment or no pigment increases, and so the overall colour of the hair changes. Grey hair is the result of a large number of white

Hair with no pigment at all

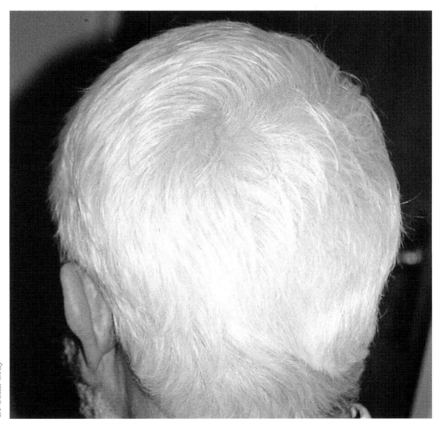

Dr John Gray

hairs growing amongst the naturally coloured hairs. The amount of 'grey' hair is often described as a percentage of the whole head. For example, if half of the hairs are white and half are still naturally pigmented, the hair is described as being '50% grey'.

Describing colour

Naturally pigmented hair colours are often simply described as being blonde, red, brown or black. Although these descriptions are adequate for general use, they are not precise enough for professional hair colouring. The International Colour Chart (ICC) was developed so that hair colours could be accurately identified and described – both the *natural* hair colour and the *desired* or 'target' hair colour.

Each hair colour is described in levels of depth and tone. Depth refers to how light or dark the colour is. This is determined by the intensity of the pigments in the hair. Tone refers to the colour that is seen. This is determined by the combination of different pigments present.

The different shades of colour are numbered, starting with 1 for black through to 10 for lightest blonde. Additional numbers are then added to each shade to identify the huge range of tones that are possible.

The International Colour Chart

Colour	Depth	Colour	Tone
1/0	blue-black	–/0	natural
2/0	black	–/1	special ash
3/0	dark brown	–/2	cool ash
4/0	medium brown	–/3	honey gold
5/0	light brown	–/4	red/gold
6/0	dark blonde	–/5	purple
7/0	medium blonde	–/6	violet
8/0	light blonde	–/7	brunette
9/0	very light blonde	–/8	pearl ash
10/0	extra light blonde	–/9	soft ash

Hair colourants

Colouring is the general term used to describe the various techniques and processes that are used to change hair colour. It is achieved through a process that adds colour pigments to the hair in the form of natural or synthetic dyes.

The history of hair colouring goes back many thousands of years. People have changed their natural hair colour for many reasons, sometimes to meet the requirements of a religion or society, but most often to express their individuality and create a look that they like.

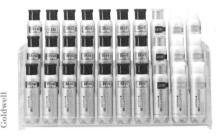

Goldwell

Colouring products

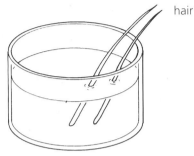

hair

small beaker

No reaction – hair and selected product are compatible

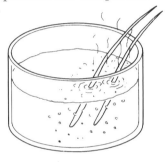

Reaction (between chemicals in product and chemicals already on hair) – hair and product are incompatible

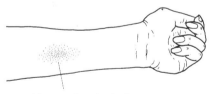

skin reaction to test

Skin test for an allergic reaction

Colourants used

Over the years, various methods and lotions have been used to change the colour of hair. Around 2000 years ago the Egyptians used the powdered leaves of the henna plant to colour hair red. The Romans used a mixture consisting largely of ash, sodium bicarbonate and lime to lighten the hair. Many other natural and artificial ingredients have been used, with varying degrees of success. In the early 1800s, however, hydrogen peroxide was discovered, and more modern methods of colouring were established. Today, most hair colourants are derived from either vegetable or mineral extracts.

Vegetable colourants

Vegetable colourants are made from the flowers or stems of different plants, such as henna. For example, camomile, made from the flowers of the camomile plant, is used to brighten light blonde hair.

Mineral colourants

Mineral colourants are made from either metallic dyes or aniline derivatives. Metallic dyes are used to coat the surface of the hair, and are sometimes used in hair colour restorers, though they are not often used in the salon.

Special care must be taken to identify whether mineral colourants have been used as *metallic dyes are incompatible with hydrogen peroxide*, and peroxide forms part of many hairdressing products used in colouring, bleaching and perming. An incompatibility test should be carried out when the use of metallic dyes is suspected.

Aniline derivatives

Aniline derivatives are synthetic dyes made from ingredients found in crude oil. They are used in most modern hair colourants and are known as para dyes.

These types of dye can cause a skin reaction, so a skin test is carried out before they are applied.

Health & Safety

Follow the manufacturers' instructions for testing carefully. Do not apply products containing para dyes to a client who has had a positive reaction to a skin test. Do not apply products containing hydrogen peroxide to hair that has produced a positive reaction to an incompatibility test.

Make sure that you keep a record of the skin test and its results and a record of your consultation and the client's responses in case of problems.

Ask the client to check their responses and sign to confirm they are correct.

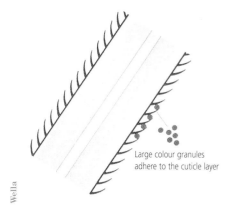

Wella

Temporary hair colouring

Large colour granules
adhere to the cuticle layer

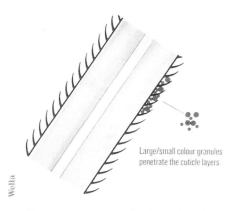

Wella

Semi-permanent hair colouring

Large/small colour granules
penetrate the cuticle layers

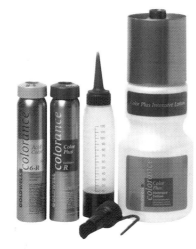

Goldwell

**Permanent hair colouring
products**

Groups of colourants

Hair colourants are usually grouped according to how long they remain on the hair.

Temporary colourants

Temporary colourants are available as lotions, mousses, and creams, sprays gels, and so on. They contain large colour molecules which *coat* the hair cuticle. They do not penetrate into the hair cortex or affect the natural hair colour, though some temporary colours may be absorbed if the hair is very porous. Temporary colours remain on the hair until they are washed off.

Semi-permanent colourants

Semi-permanent colourants are available in several forms, though they are usually applied as a cream or rinse. Most are pre-mixed, but some have to be mixed before they are used, so it is important to read the manufacturer's instructions carefully.

Semi-permanent colourants deposit their colour molecules in the hair cuticle, and also in the outer part of the hair cortex: the molecules are smaller than those found in temporary colours. This means that the semi-permanent colour molecules are more difficult to remove, so the colour lasts longer, gradually fading as the hair is washed. The colour lasts for between six and eight washes, depending upon the condition and porosity of the hair.

Semi-permanent colourants are not suitable for covering large percentages of white hair.

Quasi-permanent colourants

Quasi-permanent colourants are nearly permanent. They last longer than semi-permanent colours, but not as long as permanent colours. (The prefix 'quasi' means 'almost but not quite'.)

This type of colourant is more effective at covering white hair than are semi-permanent colourants, and can last for up to 12 weeks.

Permanent colourants

Permanent colourants, sometimes called permanent tints, are available in the form of creams and liquids, and come in a wide variety of shades and tones. They can cover white hair and naturally pigmented hair to produce natural or fashion shades, which can be very vibrant if the client so desires.

The colour molecules in permanent colourants are much smaller than those found in temporary and semi-permanent colourants: they pass easily into the hair cortex. Most permanent colourants are mixed with hydrogen peroxide. This oxidises the hair's natural pigments, causing them to combine with the molecules in the colourant and form larger molecules which become permanently trapped in the cortex.

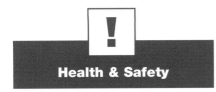

Before using permanent colourants, including toners, you must perform a **skin test**.

Permanent hair colouring

Wella

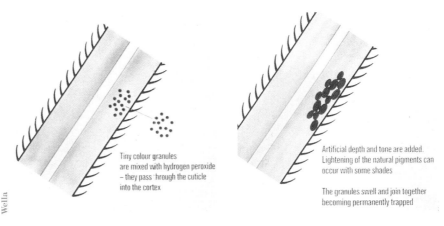

Tiny colour granules are mixed with hydrogen peroxide – they pass through the cuticle into the cortex

Artificial depth and tone are added. Lightening of the natural pigments can occur with some shades

The granules swell and join together becoming permanently trapped

Permanent colourants stay in the hair until the hair grows out, when the hair's natural pigmentation will again become visible. This regrowth must be re-coloured if the client wishes to keep his hair the desired colour.

Bleaching

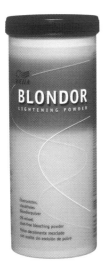

Wella

Hair bleaching/lightening product

Bleaching is the process used to make the hair colour lighter when hair colourants are not strong enough to be effective. Bleaches are available in the form of liquids, oils, creams, gels and powder.

Bleach requires a ready supply of oxygen to work. Mixing the bleach with the correct strength of hydrogen peroxide provides this. Bleach is *alkaline*. It causes the hair shaft to swell and the cuticles to lift, allowing the bleach to enter the hair cortex, where the oxygen reacts with the colour pigments, leaving them colourless.

The eumelanin pigment, which produces the colours black and brown, is the first to be affected; then the pheomelanin pigment, which gives red and yellow colours. Pheomelanin is more difficult to alter, so it becomes more noticeable as the eumelanin is lightened, sometimes making the hair appear yellow or 'brassy'. As the bleaching process proceeds, the hair gradually becomes lighter until at some point it stops getting any lighter.

The actual colour that can be achieved by bleaching depends on the proportions of eumelanin and pheomelanin in the hair. Some

Tip

When colouring, bleaching or toning, remember to take into account the temperature of the salon. A warm room will *reduce* processing time, while a cold room will *increase* processing time.

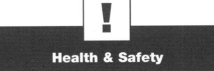

Too much bleaching will destroy the hair structure. Do not bleach hair that is in poor condition. Always avoid overlapping sections or combing bleach through hair that has been previously bleached. Before starting, process a strand of hair with a **strand test**.

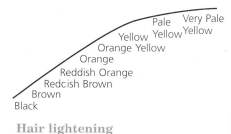

Hair lightening

natural shades, such as light brown and blond, can simply be bleached to the correct light shade. Most dark shades, however, need a toner applied to neutralise any remaining yellow. There are special toners made specifically for lightened hair, or diluted temporary, semi-permanent or permanent colourants may be used instead.

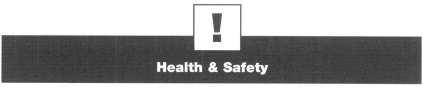

Take care not use too strong a solution of peroxide. Strong solutions can easily damage the hair structure and burn the skin. Avoid the bleach coming into contact with your own or your client's skin.

Tip

Always read the manufacturers' instructions and follow them carefully when using colouring and bleaching products.

Bleached blond hair

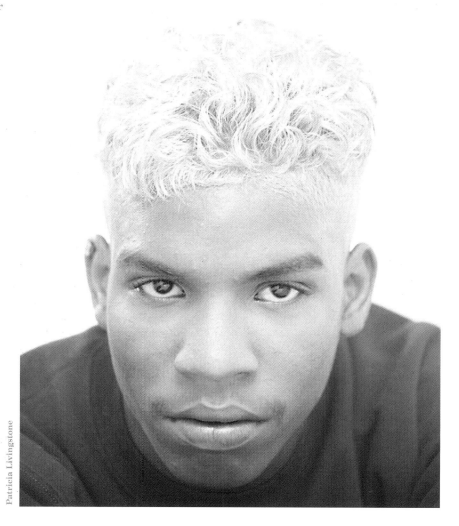

Patricia Livingstone

Consultation for colouring men's hair

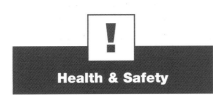

Health & Safety

You must carry out a thorough consultation to ensure that you identify any adverse conditions of the hair or skin. It is particularly important to establish whether a suspected infection or infestation is present, to check for an allergic reaction to para dyes, and to check whether the skin is inflamed, cut or grazed. If any of these conditions is present, you must not colour the hair. (This area is also covered in Chapter 2, 'Client care for men'.)

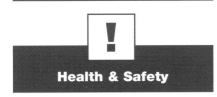

Health & Safety

Clean all tools thoroughly after use to ensure that they are ready for the next client.

Tip

Treat the hair gently after permanent colouring and especially after bleaching, particularly when drying it into style.

Tip

More detailed technical information on colouring, for both men and women, is provided in other books within the HABIA/Thomson Learning series.

Most of the principles and techniques for colouring are the same for both men's and women's hair. What differs in men's colouring is how the techniques are used to create the effects and looks that men like.

The choice of correct colouring method, product and processing time for each client relies on careful consideration of many different factors. Here are some of the critical factors that must be considered when colouring hair.

- Identify the client's requirements; then advise him on suitable styles, colouring methods and products.
- Look carefully for signs of broken skin or any abnormalities on the skin or hair.
- Determine whether the hair is fine, medium or coarse.
- Consider the client's current style and haircut, together with your client's age and lifestyle.
- If the client is a regular colouring client, refer to his record card for details of previous work.
- Determine the condition of the hair. Has it been previously chemically treated? Is the hair dry, damaged or porous?
- Carry out tests, as required.

Remember that for any client, having one's hair coloured is a major decision. For a man it can be especially so. Always discuss your client's requirements with him and establish why he wants his hair coloured and what he is expecting. Before commencing work, determine whether temporary, semi-permanent, quasi-permanent or permanent colouring is the correct solution for his needs.

Carefully explain what is involved in the type of colouring selected. Describe the benefits that your client can expect, and what after-care will be required. Here are some important things for you to cover:

- Your client may not be familiar with the type and range of colouring products that are available, so you will need to explain the benefits and features of each of them to him.
- Advise your client of the time colouring takes and the costs that are involved. Before you begin work, make sure that he agrees the course of action to be taken and check that there is no misunderstanding.
- Make sure your client knows how long each type of colour lasts, especially if the results will be permanent!
- Make sure that you prepare a record card for each client and note all details of the service accurately for future reference.
- After the colour, advise the client on how to manage his hair at home. The advice will differ depending upon the type of colour used. Hair that has been permanently coloured, and especially hair that has been bleached, will require careful handling and conditioning. Some manufacturers provide after-care information leaflets that you can give to clients.

Colouring in men's hairdressing

Men are often unaware of the benefits that colouring can bring, so they do not consider colouring services. Sometimes men are deterred from having their hair coloured because the colouring results they see displayed appear too feminine. At other times it is the service itself that acts as a deterrent, as some men find the colouring process embarrassing, particularly if it is carried out in full view of those passing by the salon.

Here are some examples of how you can introduce men to the benefits of colouring and encourage them to consider colouring services when these are the best solution for their requirements.

- Describe how colouring can provide added depth, tone and texture to enhance your client's new haircut or make his old hairstyle more interesting.
- Display examples of how colouring has been used in men's hairdressing, and especially those that illustrate how colouring can create and enhance masculine looks. Use examples of such looks to support the client consultation.
- Wherever possible, avoid using brightly coloured capes and gowns, as these may embarrass the client.

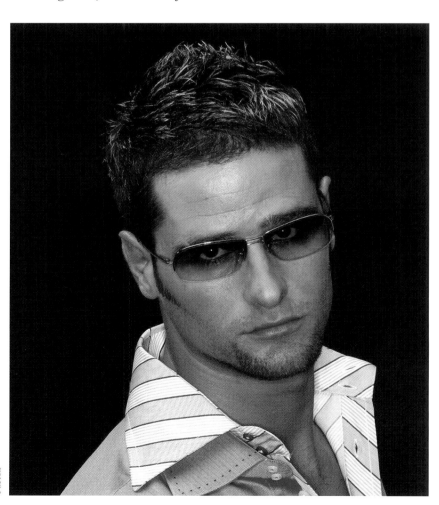

Forfex

● Carry out colouring services in areas of the salon designed for that purpose, and not in areas where other clients are only having haircutting services. Do not seat colouring clients where they can be seen by passers by.

Examples of colouring in men's hairdressing

Most men who have their hair coloured prefer the results to appear natural. Indeed, most men's colouring is carried out to enhance the haircut, and the colouring effects are often quite subtle. Full head colouring is sometimes used, but partial hair colouring, such as highlights or lowlights, is more popular with most men.

A wide range of techniques and equipment may be used to partially colour hair, including wrapping hair in caps, foil or other packages, or simply applying the product onto the selected section of hair with a brush or comb.

Partial colouring is particularly useful for defining the movement and texture within a haircut, and is often preferred by clients who have longer hair on the top and short hair at the back and sides, especially for styles that are dressed straight back on the top. Colouring can also break up solid shapes, making the hair appear more disconnected and so more interesting.

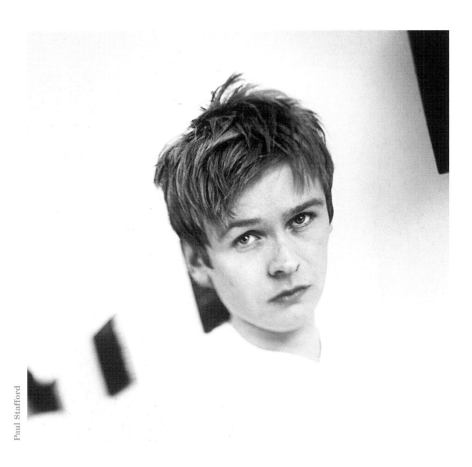

Paul Stafford

Vibrant hair colour

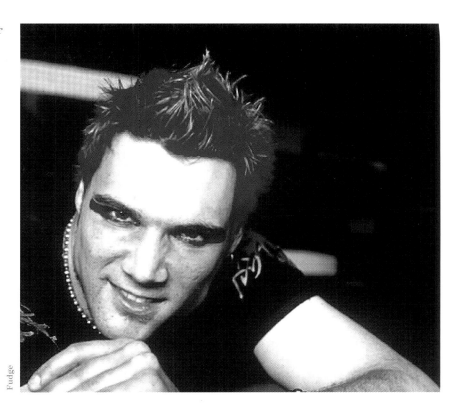

Fudge

Men generally want their hair to look as natural as possible, so vibrant coloured effects are not often required. You need always to take account of the requirements of each individual client.

The following examples show how colouring can be used to enhance some common looks. In each case the colours may be lighter or darker than the client's natural base to create either highlights or lowlights. The actual choice of colour is dependent on the requirements of each client.

Slicing

Slicing is good for defining movement on layered hair.

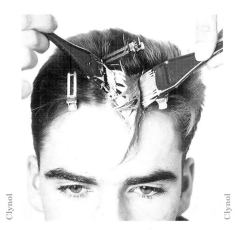

Clynol

Applying slices of colour to a selected section of hair

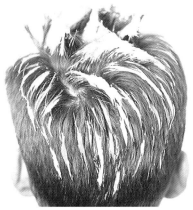

Clynol

The completed application

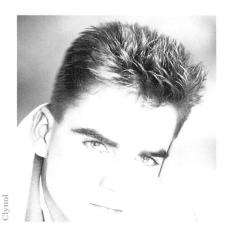

Clynol

The finished effect

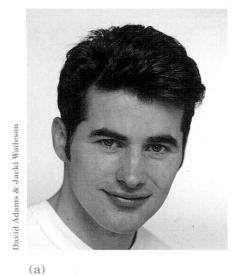

(a)

Stippling

Stippling is a development of the slicing technique. It is good for enhancing textured effects in disconnected haircuts, and for defining movement.

1   Apply barrier cream to the forehead. Place the foil on top (b).
2   Take slices across the fringe area, applying lightener as you proceed (c, d). To achieve the stippling effect, apply the lightener to a paddle brush, and brush it onto the hair (e, f). Do not overdo this, or the effects will be too solid.
3   Allow the lightener to develop, then remove it by shampooing (g).

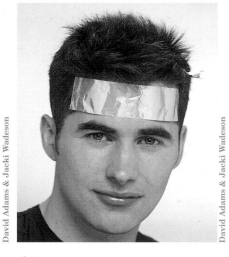

(b)

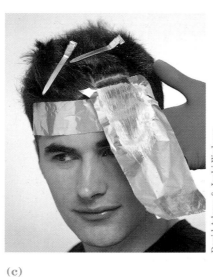

(c)

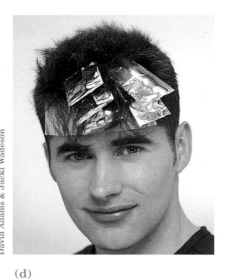

(d)

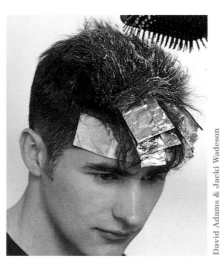

(e)

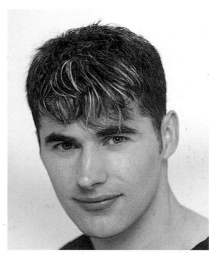

(f)

(g)

4 Using a brush, apply the colourant to the pre-lightened hair (h, i).

5 Apply colourant to the rest of the head, straight from the bottle.

6 Allow the product to develop (j), then shampoo, condition and style the hair, as required (k).

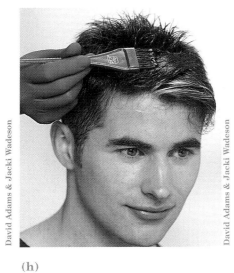

(h)

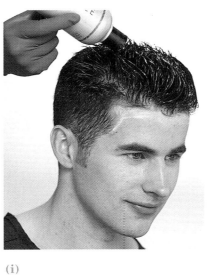

(i)

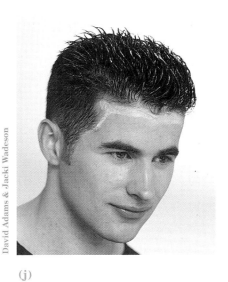

(j)

(k) The finished effect

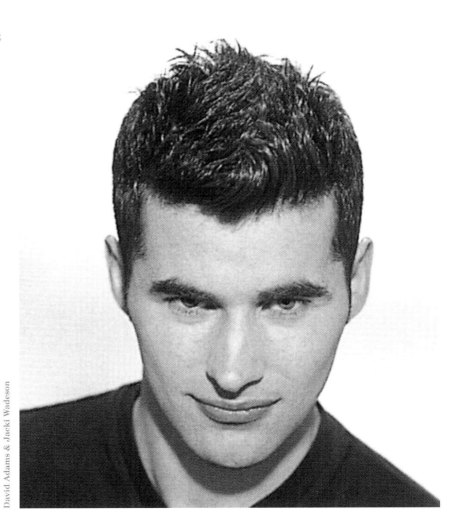

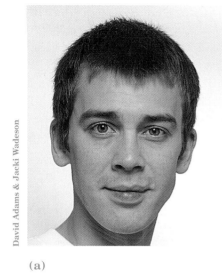

(a)

Polishing

Polishing – sometimes called shoeshine colour – is often used to create movement and texture through the ends of short layered hair.

1   Mist the hair lightly with hairspray, and blow-dry it to make the hair stand up (b).
2   Apply the first colour to a foil, using a brush (c).
3   Lightly wipe the foil across the hair, to apply colour to the ends only (d).
4   Continue applying colour over the whole of the top of the head (e).
5   Apply the second colour to the foil (f).
6   Apply the second colour, as before (g).

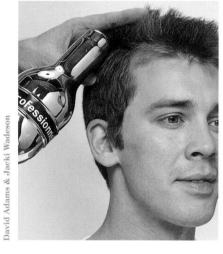

(b)

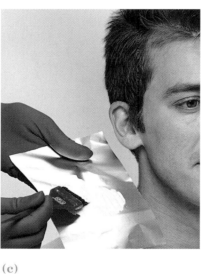

(c)

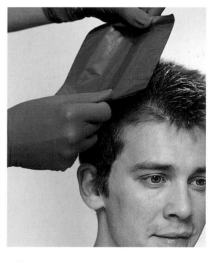

(d)

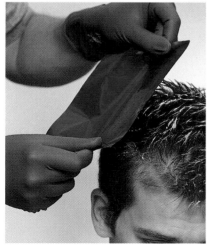

(e)

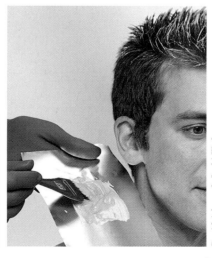

(f)

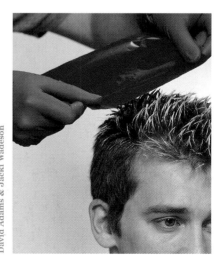

(g)

7 Allow the product to develop, then shampoo, condition and style the hair, as required (h).

(h) The finished effect

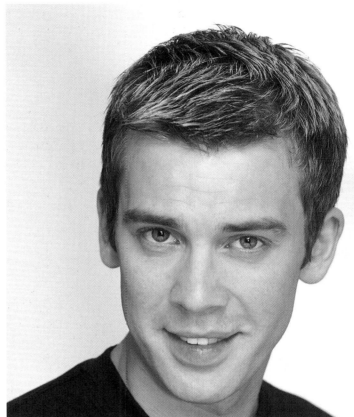

David Adams & Jacki Wadeson

Alternate final look

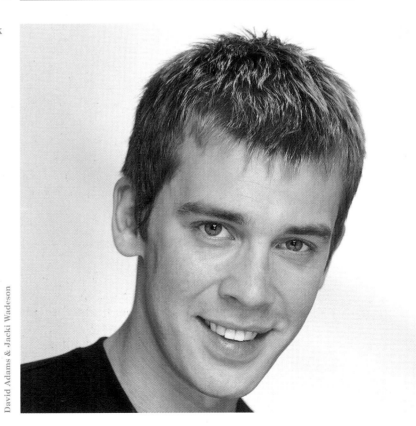

David Adams & Jacki Wadeson

Health and safety

It is important to consider health and safety when colouring hair because of the risks associated with using chemicals and the risk of damaging the skin. Here are some important health and safety factors that you must consider when providing colouring services.

Avoid infection

- If the client has any cuts or abrasions on his head, or you suspect that an infection or infestation is present, you must not carry out the colouring service.
- Use only clean tools and equipment.

Work safely with chemicals

- Always handle, use and store chemicals with care, and in accordance with the manufacturers' instructions.
- Protect your hands when using chemicals.
- Follow the manufacturers' instructions for testing, particularly for skin testing and incompatibility testing.
- Keep accurate records of skin test results and your consultation with clients for colouring services. Ask clients to check and sign their responses to confirm they are correct.
- Dispose of used chemicals in accordance with the manufacturers' instructions, salon policy, and local authority regulations.
- Check your salon's COSHH list of hazards to find out how to use products carefully.

Be prepared for accidents

- Make sure that you know the whereabouts of your salon's first-aid kit.
- Keep yourself up to date with your salon's first-aid and accident procedures.
- Take care not to splash colouring products onto the client's skin or clothes, or surrounding areas.

Activities

1   Visit local barber's shops, unisex and women's salons, and use the Internet to research colouring in men's and women's hairdressing. Find out what types of colours and effects are most popular for each. Compare your findings to identify how men use colouring services and consider how this information might help your barber's shop offer colouring services. You can then make recommendations to your manager. This activity may be combined with the similar activity in Chapter 8, 'Perming men's hair'.

2 Use the Internet and magazines to find images that show how colouring is used in men's hairdressing. Produce a style book that can be used during consultation with the clients in your salon. Remember to get permission from your manager first. This activity may be combined with the similar activity in Chapter 8, 'Perming men's hair'.

3 Practise your colouring techniques on a mannequin head or block until you can work quickly and neatly. Only then should you process the colour to become familiar with the effects. Make sure you do this before you work on clients.

4 Make a list of all the information you think should be recorded about clients relating to colouring services. Research the different record cards available at local wholesalers and use the Internet to compare them with your list. Design a new record card that includes all the most relevant information. Compare this against your salon's record card and note any differences. Recommend any improvements to your manager and be prepared to explain your reasons. This activity may be combined with the activity in Chapter 8, 'Perming men's hair'.

Check your knowledge

1 Why do we see a red object as being red?

2 What is the name of the natural pigment in the hair?

3 What effect can artificial light have on how we see colours?

4 Describe the International Colour Chart.

5 Which colour is opposite red on the colour circle?

6 Why is it important to carry out a skin test before certain colouring services?

7 What are the reasons for carrying out an incompatibility test?

8 What are the changes that take place in the hair structure during the permanent colouring process?

9 How long do quasi-permanent colours last?

10 List two types of temporary colourant.

11 Describe the changes that take place in the hair structure during the bleaching process.

12 List two types of bleach used in hairdressing.

13 State the most commonly used oxidant in colouring.

14 List seven factors that must be considered when colouring hair.

15 List three ways of encouraging men to take up colouring services.

16 State one technique that is suitable for enhancing textured effects in men's haircuts.

17 What action should be taken if the results of a skin test are positive?

18 How should you dispose of used colouring chemicals?

Perming men's hair

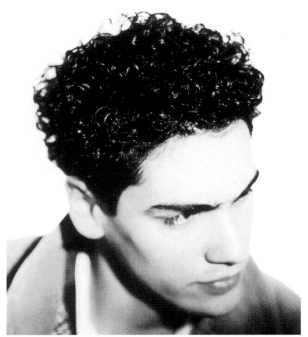

8

Vidal Sassoon

Learning objectives

Perming is the term used to describe the physical and chemical process used to change straight hair into curls or waves. Traditionally, perming has not often been required as a service in the barber's shop, so few barbers developed or offered perming services. Perming has featured in some fashionable men's looks, such as the 'curly' looks that were popular in the 1980s, but it was mostly women who requested perming services. Today, most men still do not have their hair permed, but some men have recognised that perming can provide additional volume and control and enable them to maintain looks that would otherwise be difficult to achieve.

This chapter is designed to provide an insight into how perming can be used in men's hairdressing. If you are new to perming and intend to become expert, you will need to undertake more detailed studies of the principles and techniques of perming, which are mostly the same for both men and women. Detailed technical information on perming can be found in other books within the HABIA/Thomson Learning series.

Here are some of the topics covered in this chapter:

- **the basic principles of perming and neutralising**
- **consultation for perming men's hair**
- **perming in men's hairdressing**

The basic principles of perming and neutralising

Before reading this section it may be helpful if you read Chapter 2, 'Client care for men'.

Perming, also known as permanent waving, is a technique used to change straight hair into curly or wavy hair. It is achieved through a physical and chemical process that is applied to hair that has been wound around formers, such as perming rods or curlers. The shape, size and position of the formers determine the shape and size of the curls or waves that will be produced.

Permed curls and waves are permanent: unlike those produced in blow-styling, they will not straighten out when the hair absorbs water from the atmosphere. Indeed, permed curls and waves remain in the hair until they grow out, when the hair will need to be permed again if the client wishes to retain the style.

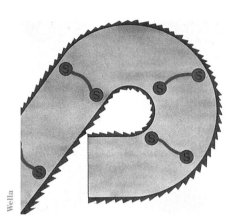

Disulphide bridges

Over the years various methods have been used to permanently curl hair. The Egyptians curled hair by winding it around sticks, which were then coated in clay and baked in the sun. In the early 1900s heat was used in hot perming systems, but this process often left the hair dry and damaged. In the 1940s cold perming or cold waving systems were introduced. Initially these too were very harsh, but today cold perms are much kinder to the hair and cold perming is now the most popular method of perming.

In the past, most cold perming lotions were alkaline. These produce good results and are particularly suitable for perming strong, coarse hair, although they may roughen the hair cuticle. Acidic perming lotions have also been popular, especially for use on dry and weaker hair, because their effects tend to be more gentle. However, more recently some ingredients in acid-balanced perms have appeared to cause skin irritation, and most manufacturers have replaced acid perms with perms that have a low alkaline content. These have a pH of about 7.1 and are often called 'pH balanced perms'.

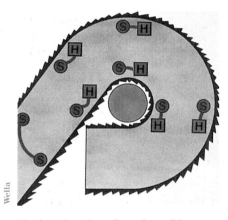

Reduction involves breaking existing disulphide bridges

The perming and neutralising process

The cold perming process consists of two key stages:

- reduction
- oxidation

Reduction

Most of the strength in hair comes from chemical links within it between sulphur atoms (S): these are called disulphide bridges. In the first stage in perming, perm lotion is used to split these, with the addition of hydrogen (H). This process is called reduction.

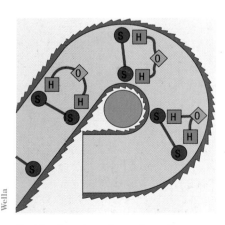

Oxidation involves forming new disulphide bridges

Following reduction, the hair is soft and pliable, and can be moulded to a new shape. The shape is determined by the rod or curler being used.

Perms and neutralisers

Wella

Oxidation

In the second stage of the perming process, the perm lotion is rinsed from the hair and a neutralising agent is applied, which stops the reduction. This process is called oxidation, neutralising or normalising. Oxygen (O) from the neutraliser combines with hydrogen in the hair, releasing water (H_2O) and forming *new* disulphide bridges. The positions of the new bridges depend on the way the hair has been moulded by the formers. When the neutraliser is rinsed away, the new bridges fix the hair in its new shape.

The most commonly used neutraliser, or oxidant, is hydrogen peroxide (H_2O_2): others include sodium bromate and potassium bromate.

Tip

Always read the manufacturer's instructions carefully.

Consultation for perming men's hair

The principles and techniques for perming men's and women's hair are mostly the same. What is different is how the techniques are used to create the effects and looks that men like.

The choice of the correct perming method, the correct lotion, and the correct processing time for each client relies on careful consideration of many different factors. Here are some of the critical factors that must be considered when perming hair.

- Identify the client's requirements, then advise him on suitable styles, perming methods and products. Determine the types of curl or waves required to achieve the chosen style, and agree the final effect to be achieved.
- Look carefully for signs of broken skin or any abnormalities on the skin or hair.
- Determine whether the hair is fine, medium or coarse.
- Consider the client's current style and haircut, particularly the hair length, together with your client's age and lifestyle.
- If the client is a regular perming client, refer to his record card for details of previous work.
- Determine the condition of the hair – is the hair dry, damaged or porous?
- Carry out tests, as required. Do not carry out the perm if there is a positive reaction to an incompatibility test. See page 139 for information on this test.

Tip

Ensure you always make a record of the products and items you have used for each client, so that future services can be carried out more easily.

Remember that for any client, having a perm is a major decision: for a man it can be especially so. Always discuss your client's requirements with him and establish why he wants a perm and

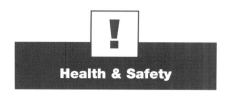

Health & Safety

You must carry out a thorough consultation to ensure that you identify any adverse conditions of the hair or skin that may be present. It is particularly important to establish whether a suspected infection or infestation is present, or if the skin is inflamed, cut or grazed. If the client has any of these conditions, you must not perm the hair. (Health and safety is covered more fully in Chapter 2, 'Client care for men'.)

what he is expecting. Before starting work, make sure that perming is the correct solution for his needs. Carefully explain what is involved in perming and describe the benefits that he can expect and what after-care will be required.

Here are some important things for you to cover.

- Your client may not be familiar with the range of perms that are available, so you will need to explain their benefits and features to him.
- Advise your client of the time perming takes and the costs that are involved. Make sure that the client agrees the course of action to be taken and that there is no misunderstanding before you commence work.
- Make sure your client understands that perming is *permanent* – the results can last for many months!
- Make sure that you prepare a record card for each client and accurately record all details of the service, for future reference.
- After the perm, advise the client on how to manage the perm at home – the hair should not be shampooed for about two days and must be handled gently. Some manufacturers provide after-care information leaflets that you can give to clients.

Perming products

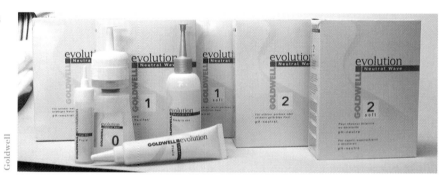

Goldwell

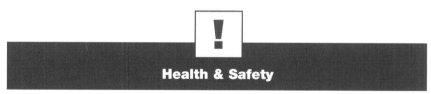

Health & Safety

Clean all tools thoroughly after use to ensure that they are ready for the next client.

Tips

Treat the hair gently after perming, especially when drying it into style. The perm may relax if you handle it too roughly.

More detailed technical information on perming for both men and women is provided in other books within the HABIA/Thomson Learning series.

Perming in men's hairdressing

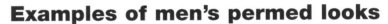

Men are often unaware of the benefits that perming can bring, so they do not consider perming services. Perming can provide added volume and control which many men would find beneficial as it would enable looks to be achieved that would otherwise be difficult. It can also help overcome specific hair problems, such as cowlicks or double crowns.

Sometimes men are deterred from having their hair permed because the perming results they see displayed appear too feminine. At other times it is the service itself that can act as a deterrent, as some men find the perming process embarrassing, particularly if it is carried out in full view of those passing by the salon.

Here are some examples of how you can introduce men to the benefits of perming and encourage them to consider perming services where these are the best solution for their requirements.

- Display examples of how perming can be used in men's hairdressing. Choose especially those that illustrate how perming can create masculine shapes. Use examples of such looks to support the client consultation.
- Wherever possible, avoid using brightly coloured perming formers, capes and gowns, as these may embarrass the client.
- Carry out perming services in areas of the salon designed for that purpose, and not in areas where other clients are only having haircutting services. Do not seat perming clients where they can be seen by passers by.

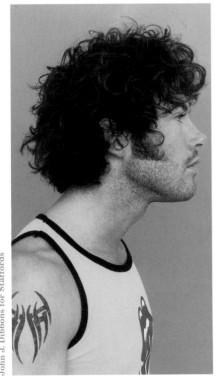

John J. Dibbons for Staffords

Examples of men's permed looks

Most men who have their hair permed prefer the curls or waves to appear natural. Indeed, most men's perming is carried out to produce volume and control to achieve a particular look: the permed curls or waves are barely visible when the hair has been dried and finished.

Partial perming, so called because only a section of the head is permed, is often more popular with men than full-head perming. Partial perming is particularly useful for clients who have long hair on the top and short hair at the back and sides, especially for styles that are dressed straight back on the top. Partial perming is also often used to provide volume or control in specific areas, though in each case the main requirement is that the permed effects appear natural.

Here are some examples of looks that may be achieved using perming.

- Perming is often best used to support the creation and maintenance of a particular look. The actual permed curls and waves are often not visible in the finished result, but they hold the blow-dried and dressed hair in place.

● Men generally want their hair to look as natural as possible, so curly perms are not often required. You need to consider the requirements of each individual client.

● Avoid producing perming results that are too round and full, as these tend to be more feminine. Remember that on most men taller, leaner shapes are more flattering.

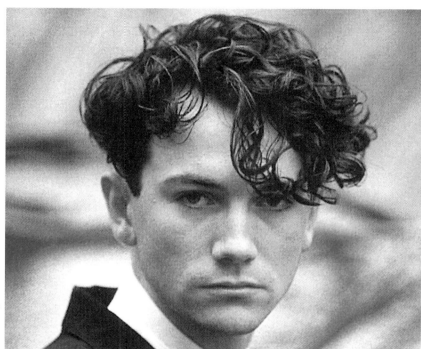

Schwarzkopf

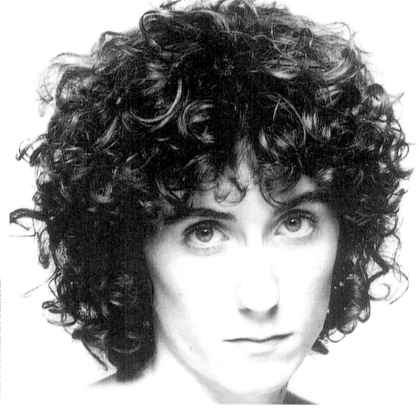

John J. Dibbens for Staffords

Health and safety

It is important to consider health and safety when perming hair because of the risks associated with using chemicals and the risk of damaging the skin. Here are some important health and safety factors that you must consider when providing perming services.

Avoid infection

- If the client has any cuts or abrasions on his head, or you suspect that an infection or infestation is present, you must not perm the hair.
- Use only clean tools and equipment.

Work safely with chemicals

- Always handle, use and store chemicals with care, and in accordance with the manufacturers' instructions.
- Protect your hands when using chemicals.
- Dispose of used chemicals in accordance with the manufacturers' instructions, salon policy, and local authority regulations.
- Check your salon's COSHH list of hazards to find out how to use products correctly.

Be prepared for accidents

- Make sure that you know the whereabouts of your salon's first-aid kit.
- Keep yourself up to date with your salon's first-aid and accident procedures.
- Take care not to splash the client's skin when applying and rinsing products.

Activities

1   Visit local barber's shops, unisex and women's salons and use the Internet to research perming in men's and women's hairdressing. Find out what types of styles and perms are most popular for each. Compare your findings to identify how men use perming services and consider how this information might help your barber's shop offer perming services. You can then make recommendations to your manager. This activity may be combined with the similar activity in Chapter 7, 'Colouring men's hair'.

2   Use the Internet and magazines to find images that show how perming is used in men's hairdressing. Produce a style book that can be used during consultation with the clients in your salon. Remember to get permission from your manager first. This

activity may be combined with the similar activity in Chapter 7, 'Colouring men's hair'.

3 Practise your winding techniques on a mannequin head or block until you can wind quickly and neatly. Only then should you process the wind to become familiar with the effects. Make sure you do this before you work on clients.

4 Make a list of all the information you think should be recorded about clients relating to perming services. Research the different record cards available at local wholesalers and use the Internet to compare them with your list. Design a new record card that includes all the most relevant information. Compare this against your salon's record card and note any differences. Recommend any improvements to your manager and be prepared to explain your reasons. This activity may be combined with the similar activity in Chapter 7, 'Colouring men's hair'.

Check your knowledge

1 Describe the changes that take place in the hair structure during the reduction process.

2 Describe the changes that take place in the hair structure during the neutralising process.

3 List two types of perming lotion.

4 What is the most commonly used oxidant in neutralising?

5 List seven factors that must be considered when perming hair.

6 List three ways of encouraging men to take up perming services.

7 What type of perming is most popular with men?

8 What are the main requirements of COSHH relating to the use of perming products?

9 Give two ways of being prepared for accidents in the barber's shop.

Scalp massage

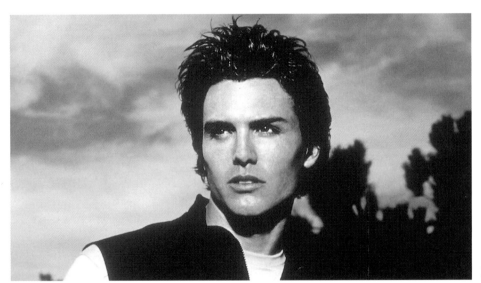

Joico

Learning objectives

Different forms of massage have been practised for thousands of years for both their psychological and physical effects. Massage involves manipulation of the skin and muscles to produce either a relaxing or invigorating sensation for the client and stimulation of the skin and underlying tissues. Various forms of scalp massage have been established to apply these effects to the head and neck for different purposes. During shampooing, massage is used to distribute and agitate the shampoo on the hair and scalp in order to remove dirt. In earlier barber's shops scalp massage was often used in services such as wet and dry shampooing, friction head massage and as part of high frequency scalp treatments.

In this chapter we will be looking at the traditional techniques used by barbers for providing scalp massage and will be covering the following topics:

- **scalp massage – the effects and benefits**
- **consultation for scalp massage**
- **scalp massage products and equipment**
- **scalp massage preparation**
- **scalp massage techniques – including effleurage, petrissage, tapotement, friction and vibro massage**
- **high frequency treatment**
- **a scalp massage routine**
- **after-care**
- **notes on health and safety**

Scalp massage – effects and benefits

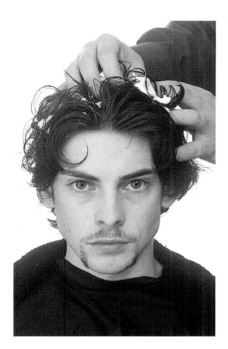

Scalp massage can be used to agitate shampoo and cleanse the hair and scalp during wet shampooing, where it also provides a pleasant and enjoyable sensation for the client. In times past many barbers would also offer dry shampooing services where a spirit-based lotion removed dirt as it was massaged into the hair and scalp, but this is rarely offered in salons today because wet shampooing is more effective. Scalp massage is usually performed with the hands, which manipulate the soft tissues of the scalp and neck. Sometimes a high frequency electrical current can be introduced to enhance the stimulating effects of the massage. A mechanical massager, more commonly called a vibro massager, can also used. Different massage techniques can be used to produce either stimulating or relaxing affects, dependent upon the client's requirements and the area to be massaged.

The anatomy of the head and neck

Before reading this section it may help you to read Chapter 2, 'Client care for men' and the section on anatomy in Chapter 12, 'Face massage'.

The basic anatomy of the head and neck and the effects that massage has on its structures and systems must be understood by the barber before providing scalp massage services.

Scalp massage

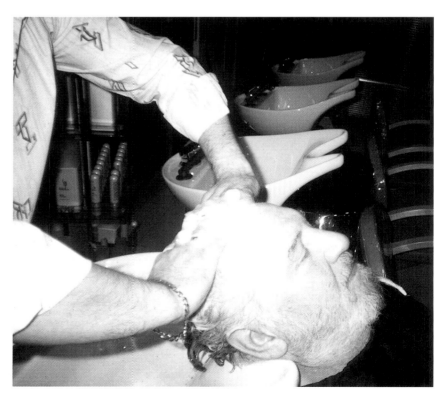

Bones of the neck and cranium

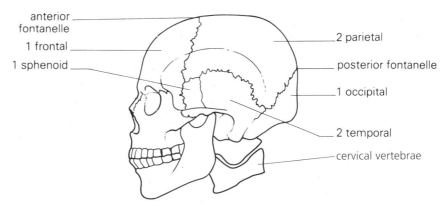

anterior fontanelle
1 frontal
1 sphenoid
2 parietal
posterior fontanelle
1 occipital
2 temporal
cervical vertebrae

- **Bones** are the foundation on which all other structures and systems are dependent. The bones of the cranium that are of particular interest in scalp massage are the frontal, sphenoid, parietal, temporal and occipital bones. On the scalp there is little tissue between the bones and the surface of the skin. In these areas you must take care to choose the right massage technique and adjust both the speed and depth of pressure to avoid causing discomfort. The bones of the neck are also important in scalp massage services and are known as the cervical vertebrae.

Muscles of the head, face and neck

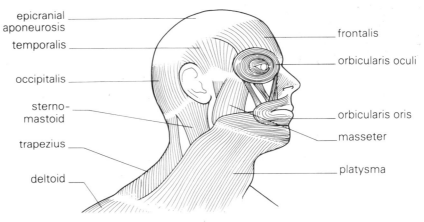

epicranial aponeurosis
temporalis
occipitalis
sterno-mastoid
trapezius
deltoid
frontalis
orbicularis oculi
orbicularis oris
masseter
platysma

- The **muscles** are interlinked with the bones and other muscles to form an integrated system. The main muscles relevant to scalp massage are the:
  - *occipital-frontalis*, a muscle that covers the front of the cranium; it enables you to lift the eyebrows, as when frowning
  - *epicranial aponeurosis* on the top of the head where the frontalis, temporalis and occipitalis muscles meet
  - *temporalis*, a muscle that connects the temporal bone with the malar and mandible bones; it enables you to close your mouth and helps with chewing
  - *occipitalis*, the muscle that covers the back of the cranium
  - *sternomastoid*, a muscle that runs behind the ears to the temporal bones and helps the head to rotate and bow
  - *trapezius*, a muscle that joins the back of the head to the shoulders; it also helps the head to rotate and bow
- **Nerves** carry messages to (and from) the brain to all parts of the body. They may be either soothed or stimulated during scalp massage, depending on the technique used.

- The **blood supply** and **lymphatic system** can both be stimulated by the application of scalp massage techniques. The main blood supply to the head is through the carotid arteries, which divide into many smaller arteries and capillaries. Eventually the capillaries rejoin to form venules and then veins, which return oxygen-depleted blood back to the heart, where it is replenished with oxygen in the lungs and returned to the arteries. The main veins from the head run down the sides of the neck and are called the jugular veins.

  The lymphatic system is made up of a network of vessels and lymph glands that closely follow the veins throughout the body. Its main functions are to remove bacteria, foreign matter and excess fluids from the tissues. Unlike the blood supply, the lymphatic system contains no pump and its contents, called lymph, are forced to move around the body by the movement of the larger muscles. Scalp massage can help to promote the flow of lymph from the head and so remove waste products and toxins from the tissues.

The effects and benefits of scalp massage

Scalp massage has many effects and benefits, including:

- increasing the supply of blood to nourish and promote healthy muscles and a healthy skin colour, called hyperaemia
- increasing the supply of blood to the hair root, called the hair papilla in order to nourish cell growth in the germinal matrix where new hair is formed
- stimulation and toning of the underlying tissues to help break down fatty deposits and improve muscle tone
- increasing the circulation of the lymphatic system to help remove waste products and toxins from the skin
- stimulation or soothing of the nerves, depending on the massage technique being used
- relaxation of the client, both physically and psychologically, thereby helping to relieve tension

Consultation for scalp massage

Before commencing a scalp massage it is important that you assess whether the client is suitable for massage. You must also establish his expectations and provide advice on the actual results that he can expect. Here are some important factors that you must consider before providing a scalp massage:

- Find out why he wants a scalp massage – is it primarily to cleanse and tone the scalp or is it for relaxation, or perhaps it's for both reasons?

- Look for any signs of broken skin, abnormalities on the skin or any other contra-indications to carrying out the massage. Remember that the contra-indications may not always show up easily, so you should ask the client if he suffers from any skin disease or skin disorder. Make sure you do this tactfully and take care not to embarrass the client.

- Examine the hair and scalp to determine whether its condition is normal, dry or greasy and establish whether any adverse conditions are present. Discuss your findings with your client and agree on the most suitable products to use.

- Consider the length and density of the hair in order to adjust the techniques and amount of product used. Manual massage can be used on any hair length and density, but mechanical massage is usually easier on shorter, layered hairstyles. On clients with less dense hair growth, such as those affected by male pattern baldness, the massage movements may have to be lighter, as the fingers are placed directly on the scalp during most of the massage. On such clients spirit-based products can quickly travel across the scalp and must be applied even more carefully.

!

Health & Safety

Do not proceed with a scalp massage if you see any contra-indications, especially any signs of broken skin, inflammation or disease. You should seek help from a senior colleague, if required and tactfully advise your client to see his doctor.

Your examination of the hair and scalp will ensure that you identify any adverse conditions that may be present. It is particularly important to establish whether a suspected infection or infestation is present, as this would prevent you from carrying out the scalp massage. (This area is covered more fully in Chapter 2, 'Client care for men'). Here are the most common contra-indications to scalp massage:

- broken or bleeding skin
- bruising, inflammation or swelling on the head or neck
- skin disorders – e.g. severe psoriasis
- eye disorders – e.g. conjunctivitis
- skin diseases – e.g. tinea capitis
- epilepsy – mechanical massage may trigger an attack and must not be used
- high blood pressure – mechanical massage can cause dizziness and nausea and must not be used

See the section on high frequency massage later in this chapter for information on the contra-indications to this form of treatment.

Scalp massage products and equipment

To provide scalp massage services you will need access to a range of products, tools and equipment.

There are many different kinds of scalp massage products available to create different effects; the correct one should be chosen to suit your client's hair and scalp condition and the affect required.

- **Products** required include treatment shampoos and conditioners, which are available for normal, dry and oily hair and scalp types, and other conditions like dandruff. Pre-blended oils, which are used as a massage medium for lubrication so that the hands slide easily without dragging. Some oils include a conditioner to improve dry hair and scalp conditions; others are scented with aromatherapy oils in order to produce relaxing or invigorating effects on the client. Spirit-based lotions, which may act as dry shampoos or as a friction tonic to promote a good blood supply, provide an antiseptic affect and create a cooling, invigorating sensation on the scalp – caused when their alcohol content evaporates. This makes the pores of the skin close and so reduces the risk of infection.

- **Equipment** required includes a vibro machine and its applicators for those who wish to provide mechanical massage to clients who enjoy the intense sensation that this technique produces. An adjustable chair should be available, which can be positioned to avoid you having to reach up or bend uncomfortably. A high frequency machine will be needed for clients requiring these treatments that stimulate and sanitise the skin.

Scalp massage preparation

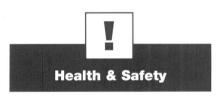

Health & Safety

Make sure that your fingernails are not too long before performing manual scalp massage, particularly when using tapotement, as long fingernails would dig into the skin.

- Carry out your consultation with the client. Look for signs of broken skin, abnormalities on the hair and scalp and any contra-indications. Determine the condition of the hair and scalp.

- Agree with your client the massage techniques and products that you will use.

- Gather together all the materials, products and equipment you will require before you begin work. Place them on a trolley so that you can work efficiently.

- The client should be gowned and a clean towel placed across his chest, tucked in at the neck. A second towel should be placed around the back over the top of the first towel.

- Your hands and nails should be clean. Make sure your nails are not too long or they will catch the client's skin. Let your client see that you have washed your hands – make it clear that you use high standards of hygiene in your work.

- Position the client at the correct height in the chair.

Preparing the hair and scalp for massage

When scalp massage is being performed in conjunction with a treatment shampoo, conditioner or spirit-based shampoo the hair is combed through before commencing. For oils and spirit-based hair friction lotions and when using high frequency equipment the client's hair and scalp should be clean and dry before the product is applied and the scalp massage carried out. See the section on high

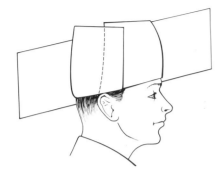

Scalp steam

frequency treatment later in this chapter for more information on using this equipment.

A scalp steam

Sometimes a scalp steam is included at the start or end of the scalp massage, where it helps to:

- open the pores and remove dirt
- open the cuticles and allow treatment products to be absorbed into the hair shaft more easily
- lubricate the scalp by stimulating the oil producing glands
- increase the flow of blood to the surface and relax the muscles to make massaging easier
- relax the client

The scalp steam can be performed with either: a hot towel – clean towels must always be used and can be prepared in a towel steamer or by soaking them in hot water – or with a steamer.

Scalp massage techniques

Tip

Before you continue with a new massage movement ask your client if the speed and pressure you are using is comfortable.

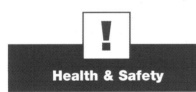

Health & Safety

Avoid using tapotement when using the high frequency equipment as the tapping movement will cause the current to jump between the client's scalp and barber's hand, causing intensive sparking and irritation. See the section on high frequency treatment later in this chapter for more information.

Before reading this section it may help you to read the section on manual massage and mechanical massage techniques in Chapter 11, 'Face massage', as the basic techniques are the same.

Scalp massage is performed using a variety of massage techniques that are used in other forms of massage. These techniques can be divided into two basic groups:

- manual massage
- mechanical massage

Manual scalp massage techniques

Effleurage is a circular, stroking movement. It is the foundation of all good massage and is used to induce relaxation, particularly at the start and the completion of the scalp massage.

Petrissage is performed through a mixture of pinching, kneading and rolling movements across the scalp. It is applied with both hands, which often work together to gently lift the skin between the fingers and thumbs, where it is squeezed, rolled and pinched with a gentle but firm pressure.

Tapotement, or percussion, is the gentle tapping of the skin with the padded part of the fingertips. On the scalp it should be applied with care because there is little underlying tissue to absorb the movements.

Friction, or vibration, is applied to the site of the nerve endings or along the path of the nerves. It is often used with friction hair tonics in scalp massage, where it enhances the stimulating effect of the tonic.

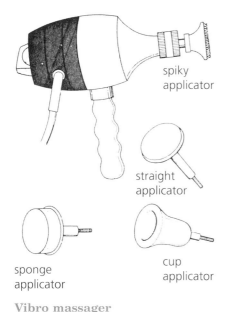

spiky applicator

straight applicator

sponge applicator

cup applicator

Vibro massager

Mechanical massage

The vibro massage is a mechanical massage technique that imitates the manual massage movements of tapotement and friction. A spiky applicator is usually used on the scalp and a rubber cup-shaped applicator on the nape area. A sponge applicator is available for use on more delicate areas, such as the temples. Vibro massage must not be used directly over delicate areas, such as around the eyes, nose or ears.

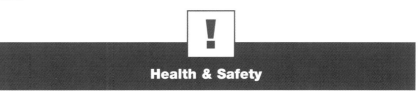

Health & Safety

Take extra care when applying massaging techniques around the temples, occipital bone and in the side of the neck. Do not use intensive tapotement or vibro techniques in these areas, as the intense movement will be very uncomfortable and may cause harm. Ensure that you use light pressure and movements on other sensitive areas.

High frequency treatment

Tip

Before you continue with a new massage movement ask your client if the speed and pressure you are using is comfortable.

A high frequency treatment is the application of an electrical current to the skin in order to stimulate the body's underlying systems and sanitise the skin surface. The high frequency electrical current is also called an alternating or oscillating current because it oscillates – moves back and forth at high speed. The speed or frequency of the oscillation is measured in hertz and in high frequency equipment the frequency of oscillation is very high, usually between 100 000 and 250 000 times, or cycles a second. This oscillating movement produces tiny vibrations on the skins surface that stimulate the skin and produce heat.

High frequency may be applied to the face, body and scalp. There are two methods:

- direct high frequency application
- indirect high frequency application

Direct high frequency application

In this method an electrode is used to apply the high frequency current to the area to be treated. The main effects of this method include:

- increased circulation of the blood supply – erythema
- increased circulation of the lymphatic system and removal of waste
- production of ozone, a gas that has a germicidal effect on the skin
- stimulation of the nerve endings
- promotion of healthy skin production

Indirect high frequency application

In this method the client holds an electrode, called a saturator whilst the area to be treated is massaged by the barber. The effects of this method include:

- increased circulation of the blood supply
- increased circulation of the lymphatic system and removal of waste
- stimulation of the sebaceous glands to help improve dry skin conditions.

Effects of high frequency on the underlying tissues

The high frequency current causes a reflex action of the blood capillaries, called vasodilatation, which leads to an increase in blood supply to the area. This nourishes the skin tissues, encourages healthy skin and hair cell production and helps healing. The sebaceous glands are also stimulated in a similar way causing them to produce more sebum and improve dry skin conditions. During the direct method of treatment tiny sparks can be created beneath the electrodes, which react with oxygen on the surface of the skin to become ionised and produce ozone. Ozone has antiseptic properties that can help improve skin blemishes. Sparking is achieved by lifting the electrode 5–10 mm away from the skin and replacing it in a gentle tapping movement. This is performed about 6–8 times in each area to be treated.

Contra-indications to high frequency treatment

Here are the most common contra-indications to high frequency treatments:

- broken or bleeding skin
- bruising, inflammation or swelling on the head or neck
- skin disorders – e.g. severe psoriasis
- skin diseases – e.g. tinea capitis (mild infections such as pustules can benefit from direct high frequency treatment)
- epilepsy – high frequency may trigger an attack and must not be used
- high blood pressure – high frequency can cause dizziness and nausea and must not be used
- migraine – high frequency may trigger an attack and should not be used
- extensive metal dental work – the metal would focus the high frequency current and be uncomfortable
- pregnancy – high frequency may cause problems for the mother and/or unborn child and must not be used

High frequency unit

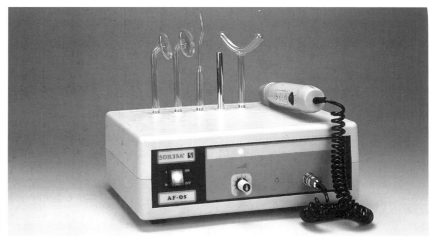

Sorisa

- chemotherapy – high frequency can cause problems and lead to dizziness and nausea
- radiotherapy – dizziness and nausea and other problems can occur
- hypersensitive skin
- heart pacemakers – high frequency equipment may interfere with the sensitive electronics in heart pacemakers and must not be used

High frequency equipment

The following equipment is needed to perform high frequency scalp massage treatments:

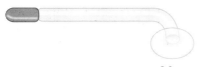

ø 30 mm

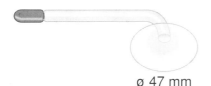

ø 47 mm

Mushroom electrodes

- *A high frequency unit*
- *Electrodes* There are glass electrodes and a metal electrode. Each has a metal cap that slots into the electrode holder that allows the electric current to pass into the electrode. Glass electrodes contain a small amount of gas, usually air, mercury vapour or neon, which allows the current to pass down the electrode. Glass electrodes glow when in use – the different gases produce different colours:

  – air – violet

  – mercury vapour – blue

  – neon – orange

Electrodes are available in a variety shapes and sizes for treating different areas and producing different effects. The following electrodes are readily available and are used in various ways in scalp treatments:

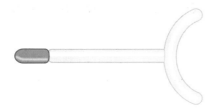

Horseshoe electrode

- *Mushroom electrode* – available in different sizes; the smaller the size the more intense the effect. Used around the hairline and to create sparking.
- *Horseshoe electrode* – shaped to the contours of the neck and used in the nape area.

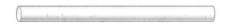

Saturator electrode

- *Saturator electrode* – held by the client whilst the barber performs the scalp massage.

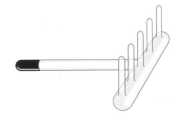

Rake electrode

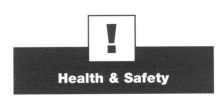

Health & Safety

Do not use high frequency equipment near water because of the risks of electrocution.

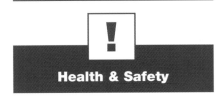

Health & Safety

The electrodes must be effectively cleaned and sanitised after use. They should be cleaned with disinfectant and placed in a sterilising cabinet for over 20 minutes – make sure they are turned during the process to ensure all sides are sanitised.

● *Rake electrode* – combed through the hair to create a series of more intense sensations.

Preparation for high frequency scalp application

1   Check the client's record card and carry out a consultation (this may be performed as part of the consultation for the complete scalp massage)

2   Remove metal items from your own hands and wrists

3   Sanitise your hands

4   Ensure that your client is correctly gowned and protected and his hair prepared – hair should be clean and dry and combed back. Ask the client to remove any metal items from the treatment area or from their hands and wrists if using the indirect method of application

5   Check that the equipment is in good working order and appears safe to use

6   Select a suitable electrode for the application method and treatment area and slot it into the electrode holder

7   Explain the procedure to the client

8   Set the current intensity to zero. Switch on the machine and place the electrode to be used against your own skin. Increase the current intensity until a buzzing sound is heard and a slight sensation is felt. Return the current intensity to zero, switch off the machine, sanitise the electrode and replace it in the electrode holder.

The high frequency application is covered in the next section.

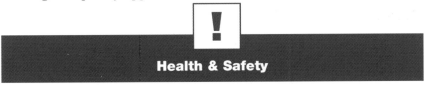

Health & Safety

Metal objects, such as watches and jewellery conduct the high frequency electrical current more easily. This focuses and intensifies the effects of the current and is uncomfortable for the client and barber. Metal items should be removed from the treatment area, or insulated if they cannot be removed, before commencing the treatment.

A scalp massage routine

There are several different ways of performing a scalp massage. The starting place, pattern of movements and method of completion are all adapted to suite the client, barber and effect required. Most barbers follow a preferred routine and use their own creativity to make the massage more pleasurable and effective. Some scalp massages include both manual and mechanical massage, whilst others use just manual massage techniques. Some manual scalp massages include a high frequency treatment, but few scalp massages use only vibro massage. Whatever massage is performed a good scalp massage will always follow these simple rules:

- Manual scalp massage should start and end with a relaxing massage movement, usually effleurage.
- The sequence of massage movements should flow logically so that the sensation created is one of continuous massage.
- Repeat each movement several times before moving on to the next area of the scalp.
- Ensure that you cover all areas of the scalp, unless your consultation has identified otherwise.
- Do not rush; your goal is to make the massage pleasant and relaxing.

The following routine is one example of how a scalp massage may be performed.

A manual scalp massage routine

1 Ensure that your client is correctly gowned and protected.
2 Prepare the hair, as required.
3 Apply a scalp steam, if required.
4 Apply sufficient massage product to lubricate the scalp and cover the hair – do not apply too much so that it overloads the skin and hair. Start at the front hairline and distribute the product around the head using effleurage.
5 Use light effleurage movements to relax the client, each hand moving in alternate directions (imagine you are drawing a zigzag pattern across the head). Work slowly and carefully to let the client become accustomed to the sensation.
6 Move the fingers back towards the temples then make small circular effleurage movements working back across the head to the crown area. Repeat this series of movements several times working up to the top of the head.
7 Slide your fingers down the back of the head and make spiralling effleurage movements with each hand down to the nape, moving back up towards the crown after each stroke.
8 Place the fingers on the front hairline. Using light pinching and squeezing petrissage movements, work back along the head to the crown. Slide the fingers back down to the temples and then work back up towards the top of the crown, using the pinching movements as before. Make sure you cover all of the head.
9 Slide back down to the nape area. Using the middle fingers of each hand make two deep, rotating petrissage movements then continue this movement up across the head and to the temples. Repeat this movement several times.
10 Slide your fingers back to the front hairline. Using your fingertips apply a very light tapping tapotement movement and work back across the head to the crown and down the back to the nape. Avoid the temples, occipital bone and side of the neck. Repeat these movements from the sides to the nape. You should develop a gentle rhythm to make the movement enjoyable.

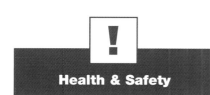

Health & Safety

Remember – your hands must be clean before you commence the scalp massage. Let your client see that they are being cleaned.

Tip

Make sure that the head is tilted back slightly if you are applying spirit-based lotions to avoid the lotion running into the client's eyes. These lotions should be applied onto the back of your hand while it is placed with the fingers splayed on the scalp, so that the lotion travels down your fingers and is spread around the head more evenly.

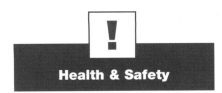

Tip

Little pressure is required when using a vibro massager on the scalp.

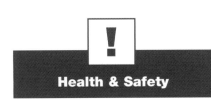

11 Complete the massage routine with gentle sweeping effleurage movements across the head and neck.

12 The hair may now be shampooed to remove excess massage oil, if required, or rinsed to remove any treatment shampoo or conditioner that may have been used and then dried and styled. If a spirit-based lotion has been used the hair can be dried and styled unless it is to be vibro massaged. The hair and scalp should be roughly dried if high frequency is to be applied.

13 Record details of the treatment given onto the client's record card, if not continuing with vibro massage or high frequency.

14 Provide after-care advice.

A vibro massage routine

Scalp massage may be completed with a vibro massager, which may be used either on its own or in conjunction with the manual massage techniques. Make sure your client desires this form of massage before using it. The vibro massager is used following the same pattern of movements as when applying manual massage techniques, but extra care must be taken. Ensure that you use light pressure and movements throughout. Avoid using it on the temples, occipital bone and in the side of the neck.

The spiky applicator is used for most scalp massage movements and can produce intense stimulating effects. The cup and sponge applicators have a more gentle and relaxing effect and should be used on the neck.

High frequency application

A scalp massage may include the use of high frequency equipment for those clients seeking the benefits of this treatment. Both direct and indirect methods of application are usually used in scalp massage, commencing with the direct method.

Direct high frequency application method

1 Prepare the high frequency unit (see the high frequency section earlier in this chapter).

2 Ensure that your client is correctly gowned, protected and prepared.

3 Switch on the mains power to the high frequency unit.

4 Ensure that the current intensity setting is at zero and switch on the machine.

5 Place the mushroom electrode in the holder and then in contact with the client's skin at the middle of their front hairline. Increase the current intensity to the desired level.

6 Move the electrode over the skin in a circular, rotary movement following the natural hairline down one side, around the ear and into the nape. Make sure that the end of the electrode remains in contact with the skin throughout. Repeat this on the other side.

7 Reduce the current intensity to zero and switch off the machine.

8 Place the rake electrode into the holder and switch on the machine.

Tip

The intensity of the current increases when it passes to the client's skin through a smaller area, e.g. turning the mushroom electrode so that the edge is in contact with the skin rather than the flat bulb part will increase the intensity of the sensation for the client. You can reduce the sparking and irritation caused when the electrode is removed or placed on the skin by spreading the current across your free hand. Simply place your free hand on the client's head and two fingers on part of the electrode before it is removed from or placed onto their skin.

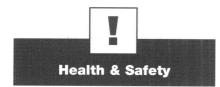

Health & Safety

Remember to avoid using tapotement when using the high frequency equipment during manual scalp massage as the tapping movement will cause the current to jump between the client's scalp and barber's hand, causing intensive sparking and irritation.

9   Place the prongs of the rake electrode on the scalp at the middle of the front hairline. Increase the current intensity to the desired level.

10 Move the electrode straight back over the scalp to the crown and down to the nape. Make sure that the prongs of the electrode remain evenly in contact with the scalp throughout.

11 Move back to the front hairline and repeat this in the adjacent section of hair. Repeat this process down the side of the head.

12 Repeat steps 9–11 on the other side of the head.

13 Reduce the current intensity to zero and switch off the machine.

Indirect high frequency application method

1   Place the saturator electrode into the holder. Check that the client is not wearing any metal items on their hands or wrists and give them a tissue to wipe their hands to remove any perspiration or grease.

2   Place the saturator electrode firmly into the client's hand and ask that they continue holding it firmly throughout the treatment.

3   Place one of your hands onto the client's head near the front hairline and begin making small effleurage movements. With the other hand switch on the machine.

4   Increase the current slowly until the client feels a slight tingling sensation at the point where your fingertips touch their scalp.

5   Place both hands on the client's head and perform a manual scalp massage following steps 5–9 of the manual massage routine earlier in this chapter. This process should last for around 10 minutes, but check that your client is comfortable and reduce the time and/or current intensity, as required. Do not perform the tapotement massage movements.

6   At the end of the massage keep one hand in contact with the scalp. Remove any massage medium from the other hand then reduce the current intensity to zero and switch off the machine and mains supply.

7   Remove the saturator from the client's hand.

8   Place your hands back on the scalp and complete the massage routine with gentle sweeping effleurage movements across the head and neck for 5 minutes.

9   The hair may now be dried and styled.

10 Record details of the treatment given onto the client's record card.

11 Provide after-care advice.

After-care

Allow the client to rest for a few moments after the scalp massage to allow their blood circulation to return to normal, especially if he has been sitting slightly reclined or he may feel a little light headed. You may offer refreshments if this is allowed in your salon. Provide advice on further treatments that may be necessary and any suitable retail products.

Health and safety

Anyone providing scalp massage services has a duty to work safely and hygienically. You must maintain high standards of hygiene in all aspects of your work and be extra careful when using electrical equipment. The following are some important factors that you must consider when providing scalp massage:

- Do not go ahead with the scalp massage if you see any contra-indications, especially any signs of broken skin, inflammation or disease. In these cases you should seek help from a senior colleague, if required and tactfully advise your client to see their doctor.

- Take extra care when applying massaging techniques around the temples, occipital bone and nape areas. Do not use intensive tapotement or vibro techniques in these areas. Use light pressure and movements on any sensitive area. Be alert to any non-verbal signs of discomfort that the client may show.

- Fingernails must not be too long or they may catch the client's skin during the massage.

- Special attention must always be paid to hygiene when providing scalp massage because your hands will be working in contact with the client's skin. Always wash your hands thoroughly before you begin work and make sure you maintain high standards of personal hygiene.

- Electrical equipment must always be handled and used with care in accordance with the manufacturer's instructions.

- *Never* use or place electric vibro machines or electrical high frequency equipment near water.

- *Do not* go near electrical equipment that is lying in water – isolate the mains power first.

- Visually check that electrical equipment is safe to use before commencing work – check that the cable has not frayed or been pulled and that the plug is not loose.

- Pay attention to the position of cables when using and storing electrical equipment.

- *Never* overload sockets by plugging too many items of electrical equipment into the same socket.

- Follow the manufacturer's instructions for the maintenance of electrical equipment.

- Only clean towels, tools and equipment should be used.

- Ensure that metal items are removed from areas to be treated with high frequency – ensure that you remove such items too!

- Make sure that you know the whereabouts of your salon's first-aid kit. Keep yourself up to date with your salon's first-aid and accident procedures.

- Re-read the section on hygiene in Chapter 2, 'Client care for men'.

Activities

1 Find out more about how electricity works and produce a simple information leaflet on high-frequency treatments. You can then use the leaflet to inform clients. Remember to check with your manager first.

2 With your colleagues, assess each others' hair and scalp condition and choose the most suitable form of scalp massage and products to use. Check your results with your manager or tutor then practise your scalp massage techniques.

Check your knowledge

1 Describe how scalp massage is usually performed.
2 List those bones of the head and neck that are of interest in scalp massage.
3 Describe the location and action of the trapezius muscle.
4 What is the name of the main blood supply to the head?
5 Explain how scalp massage affects the lymphatic system.
6 List three benefits of scalp massage.
7 Why is consultation important before scalp massage?
8 List four contra-indications to scalp massage.
9 List two products used in scalp massage and describe their effects.
10 How should the hair be prepared prior to a spirit-based hair friction scalp massage?
11 Describe a scalp steam.
12 When are effleurage massage techniques most often used?
13 What are the two things you should check with your client before continuing with a new massage movement?
14 Which vibro massage applicator is usually used on the scalp?
15 List three effects of the direct high-frequency application.
16 How is ozone produced during high-frequency treatments?
17 What type of current is produced by high-frequency equipment?
18 List eight contra-indications to high-frequency treatments.
19 Which electrode should be used around the hairline?
20 Describe the preparation requirements for a high-frequency treatment.
21 What setting should the high-frequency machine be set to at the start of the treatment?
22 Describe one important after-care requirement.
23 Why is the length of the barber's nails important in scalp massage?
24 Why is it important to place high-frequency equipment away from water?
25 List two ways of identifying whether the client is comfortable during scalp massage services.

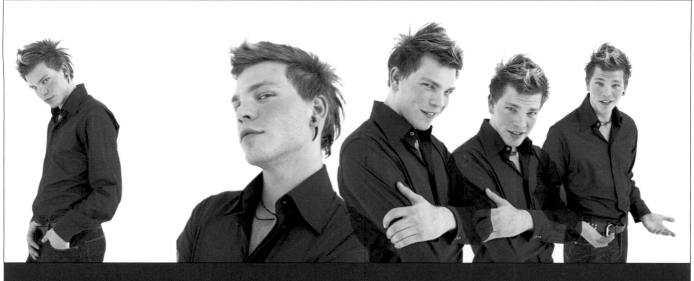

Level 3 Advanced Menswork

Advanced men's hair cutting

10

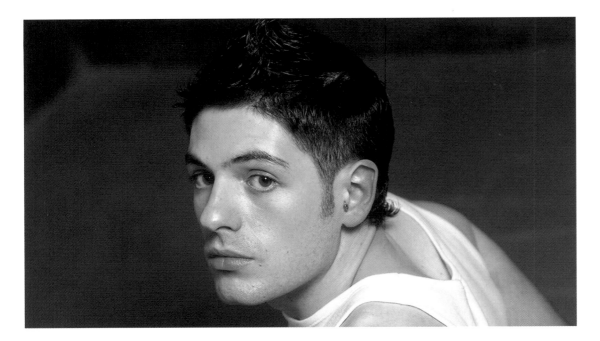

Learning objectives

All haircuts should be personalised to best suit each client's features in order to give them a more individual style or look. The haircut forms the basis of all these looks and for all the subsequent styling of the hair. Many advanced men's haircuts rely heavily on accurate cutting techniques and on an accurate finish. Other advanced haircuts demand techniques that produce highly textured effects that do not appear to conform to traditional lines and accuracy. Today's barber must have all these advanced men's hair cutting techniques at his disposal in order to create the variety of highly personalised looks that many men wear today.

In this chapter we will be looking at the techniques the barber uses for advanced men's hair cutting and will be covering the following topics:

- **factors to be considered when creating a variety of men's looks**
- **advanced cutting techniques – including tapering and texturising**
- **cutting procedures**
- **notes on health and safety**

Before reading this chapter it may help you to read Chapter 5, 'Cutting men's hair using basic techniques'.

Factors to be considered when creating a variety of men's looks

As we discovered earlier in this book, it is the haircut that forms the basis for all good hairdressing. This is especially so when creating advanced men's looks, as many of these looks would be difficult or impossible for the client to achieve at home without 'a good cut' as the foundation.

There are many similarities between basic and more advanced men's hair cutting. Often the same cutting techniques can be used and some of the looks produced have styling features that are similar to their more basic versions. Factors including facial hair, dense hair growth on the neck, male pattern alopecia (baldness) and other adverse hair and scalp conditions still have to be fully considered. Taller, less full or leaner shapes are also usually more flattering on men requiring advanced looks. But differences do exist in the overall complexity of the looks that are required and the methods that are used to achieve them.

In advanced work you will see that the principles learnt earlier about shape and form are often followed more loosely. For example, some fashionable advanced looks appear to work best by being taller and fuller! Advanced work regularly requires cutting techniques to be combined and adapted to take account of both the client's wishes and the many factors that affect the creation of the look. The client consultation is again most essential in choosing and personalising the right look for each client.

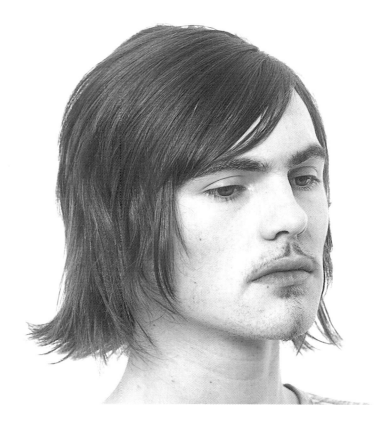

Consultation

Remember – a successful haircut will always begin with a thorough consultation! You must always make time to discuss the client's requirements and expectations with him, whether he is a new or regular client. Here is a reminder of some of the critical factors that must be considered when cutting men's hair:

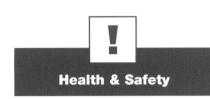

Health & Safety

You must carry out a thorough consultation to ensure that you identify any adverse conditions of the hair or skin that may be present. It is particularly important to establish whether a suspected infection or infestation is present, as this would prevent you from cutting the hair. (This area is covered more fully in Chapter 2, 'Client care for men').

- Identify the client's requirements then give him advice on suitable looks and agree the final effect to be achieved.
- Look for signs of broken skin or any abnormalities on the skin or hair.
- Look for signs of any unusual hair growth patterns and identify the natural fall of the hair.
- Determine if the hair is fine, medium or coarse.
- Is the hair growth dense or sparse – does the client have male pattern baldness?
- Is the client wearing an added hairpiece?
- Does the client have a beard or moustache? Would styling of the eyebrows enhance the look?
- Determine the features of the client's head, face and body – is the client wearing spectacles or a hearing aid?
- Establish the age of the client.
- Consider the client's lifestyle.
- Consider the style requirements of any artificial colour that has been, or will be used to determine how the haircut and colour can compliment each other.

Cutting outlines

Many men have dense hair growth that grows outside the natural hairline, particularly on the face and in the nape areas. In shorter layered looks, the haircut must always be outlined and the unwanted hair from outside the haircut outline removed or it will appear untidy and unfinished. In longer fashionable styles it can seem less important, as the longer hair may cover the hairline. Unwanted hair outside the outline should still be removed though, especially where the client may fasten his hair up in a pony tail and expose the hairline. Some outlines are cut to give a natural appearance, whilst others are created with lines so that they are obvious, and yet others are faded so that no outline is visible at all, such as the skin fade that is popular with some African-Caribbean men. The outline of a haircut is usually most noticeable in the nape, where it is known as the neckline.

Neckline shapes

These are important in men's hairdressing because the natural neck hairline is usually less well defined, as hair often grows densely on the neck. There are three basic neckline shapes that suit most men's looks and one of these is likely to be suitable for most short layered advanced men's looks:

- *squared neckline shapes* – sometimes known as a 'square cut'
- *tapered neckline shapes* – sometimes known as a 'taper cut'
- *rounded neckline shapes* – sometimes known as a 'Boston neckline'

Neckline shapes can also be cut to appear more or less natural. The correct shape and effect will meet the client's wishes and take account of the overall look and the hair growth patterns in the nape area. Longer looks below the height of a typical shirt collar usually do have more rounded neckline shapes than normally found in men's hairdressing. But heavy rounded outlines are still best avoided. Layered and textured effects usually work better, as these create movement and reduce the weight of the outline.

Stronger and more extreme looks often have styling details that are more radical. Strong, less natural outlines may be features of these types of look and in such cases the outlines can be cut to almost anywhere, or even incorporated into elaborate patterns and designs (see Chapter 14, 'Design and create patterns in hair'). Likewise, such radical details can be added to facial hair, including beards, moustaches and eyebrows to make effective contributions to the overall look required (see Chapter 13, 'Designing facial hair shapes'.

As you can see, in the same way as the principles of shape and form discussed earlier, the principles of outlining in advanced work can also be applied more loosely to achieve the correct look!

Here are some important things to remember about outlining advanced men's haircuts:

- On most men, especially with short layered looks, the haircut must still be outlined or it will appear untidy and unfinished.
- Follow the natural hairline wherever possible, particularly when outlining shorter haircuts. Avoid making unnecessary cuts into the natural hairline, especially around the ears and at the sides of the nape, unless the look requires these more radical and less natural effects.
- Many outlines appear more natural if they are gently tapered, particularly on shorter styles, in the nape and at the bottom of the sideburns.

Cutting sideburns

Sideburns are important in most men's haircuts. Usually men want sideburn shapes that are less prominent, with the emphasis on creating a natural balanced look that matches their haircut. In fashionable advanced looks sideburns are often styled into longer shapes, sometimes into points and other more elaborate designs. In each case the face shape and hairstyle should be used to determine the correct choice of sideburn shape for each client. Here are some important things to remember about cutting sideburns:

- Most men's haircuts are improved by having sideburns. Sideburns help to balance the haircut and create an attractive masculine frame to the face.

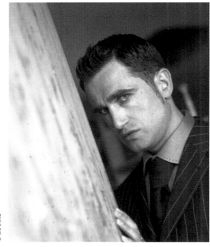
Forfex

Tip

To ensure that the sideburns are cut level place the thumb of each hand high on each sideburn. Whilst looking in the mirror slide one thumb down until the desired length is reached. Slide the other thumb down until both thumbs are level. Memorise the position of the thumbs; you can use a position on each ear as a point of reference. Now cut each sideburn to the correct length. This method can be easily adapted to establish the width of the sideburns and so obtain symmetrical shapes, even in the most elaborate sideburn designs.

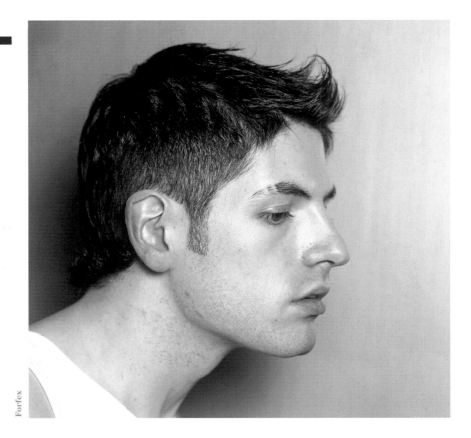

Forfex

- Avoid cutting the length of the sideburns higher than the top of the ear and into the hairline unless the look requires these more radical and less natural effects.

- Sideburns should usually be cut level, unless the look is to be asymmetric. Do not use the ears to determine the level of the sideburns, as they are not usually placed level themselves.

- Pay particular attention to where the haircut meets the sideburns and ensure that they blend together.

- Think of the haircut and sideburns as being integrated parts of one style.

Further information on cutting sideburns and facial hair and designing facial hair shapes is provided in Chapter 4, 'Cutting facial hair using basic techniques' and Chapter 13, 'Designing facial hair shapes'.

Advanced cutting techniques

Many cutting techniques, such as scissors-over-comb and clippers-over-comb are used in both men's basic haircutting and men's advanced haircutting. But differences do exist in the way that the techniques are used and in the different effects that they achieve. There are some techniques, however, which are only really used in more advanced work and these are explained in the next section.

Tapering

Tapering is used to cut the hair so that it tapers to a point. Both unwanted weight and length may be removed. It is particularly useful for blending in heavier sections of the hair, as the weight at the ends can be reduced without affecting the hair length. Here are some methods that are commonly used in tapering men's hair.

- **Scissor tapering** (sometimes called slithering) – is carried out on dry hair. It is achieved by moving the open scissor blades backwards and forwards along the hair section in a slithering, sliding movement. The blades are gently opened and closed a small amount during the movement to remove the required amount of hair. The blades must not be completely closed or the section of hair will be cut straight through.

- **Razor tapering** – sometimes just called 'razor cutting', is only used on wet hair. It is achieved by placing the razor on the hair at an angle of about 30° and then making gentle slicing movements as the razor cuts the hair. On shorter hair the section to be cut should be combed through until the comb is at least 3 cm away from the hairline. The comb is then kept in this position and the razor is placed at the correct angle on the hair about 2–3 cm down from the comb. The hair is then cut using gentle slicing movements with the razor. The razor and comb should move down the section together, remaining about 2–3 cm apart throughout.

- **Razoring** (shaving) – is sometimes used to create clean outlines and emphasise a haircut shape. It is performed with a razor, which may be either an open razor or a safety razor. Disposable blade razors are best because they are more hygienic. Electric razors are also sometimes used.

Tip

Great care must be taken when razor cutting. Do not razor cut the hair too near to the hairline or roots, as it will stick up and be very difficult to style. Always use gentle cutting actions and small movements, as the razor can quickly and easily remove too much hair if not used correctly.

Razor tapering

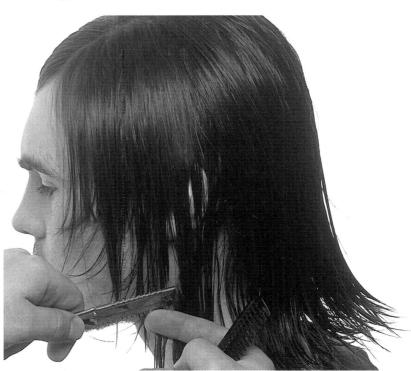

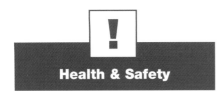

Pointcutting

Texturising

Texturising techniques are used to break up a solid mass of hair and create a more random movement and texture. Many different cutting techniques can be used to produce the varying lengths of hair that create the 'textured' effect. Most often freehand pointing, chipping, slicing and chopping actions with the scissors will produce the required effects. The razor can also be used to achieve similar effects. The hair is usually cut in the middle third of the section and towards the ends, as cutting too near the roots will make the short hairs stick out. Short layered haircuts are often texturised through the top to disconnect the shape and create a sensation of movement and energy. Freehand texturising techniques are often used in advanced work as these are able to create random effects exactly where the barber wishes.

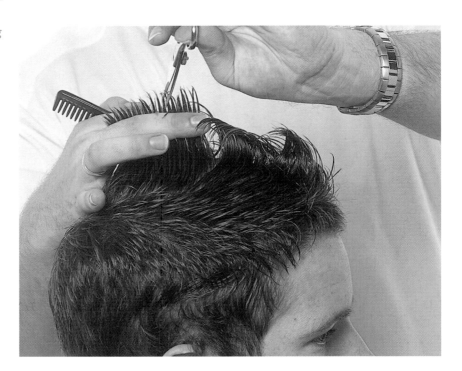

Cutting procedures

Many different cutting procedures may be followed to cut men's hair. Individual barbers will usually decide where to start and which cutting techniques to use mostly according to personal preference. In advanced cutting it is the barber's creativity and individualism that comes to the fore. The range of basic and advanced skills at his disposal enables him to choose the best technique for a specific task. Many cutting techniques can achieve similar effects and the advanced barber will combine and adapt these, as necessary, to achieve the required results. The best procedure remains one that allows the barber to work accurately and efficiently throughout the whole haircut. The following examples show how some advanced men's looks can be achieved.

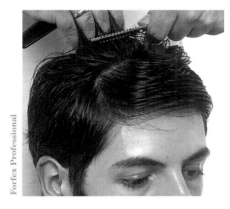

Forfex Professional

(a) Before cutting

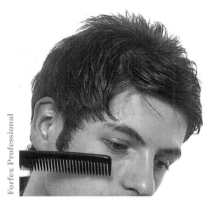

Forfex Professional

(b) Step 1

Short looks

Andrea 1 – a textured natural look

1 With the hair wet, create a parting from the top of one ear across the head to the top of the other ear and comb the hair in front of this parting forwards or across to one side. At the front of the middle panel take a section of hair up in your fingers and razor-cut this to length making sure that you create movement and texture.

2 Continue this through the crown area.

3 Move to the side and continue creating movement and texture by razor-cutting the panels down using just the toe of the razor. Use your comb as a barrier to make sure that the ears are protected. Take extra care when working against the head if using a razor without a guard fitted.

4 Dress the hair into place to judge how the shape and form is progressing.

5 Continue this technique up into the front section.

6 Remove small strands of hair around the front to break up the outline.

7 Repeat steps 5–8 on the other side and check that the shape is developing symmetrically. Continue around the back of the head.

8 Move to one side of the head. Note the required length for any sideburns that may be present, ensure they are level (see tip on page 183) and cut them to shape. Outline the sideburn and around the ears then down the sides of the nape with the tips of your scissors or with the clippers.

9 Repeat this on the other side of the head and then create the required neckline shape.

10 Shave the areas outside the haircut outlines, if required (see Chapter 11, 'Shaving').

11 Blow dry into shape and finish with wax to add definition.

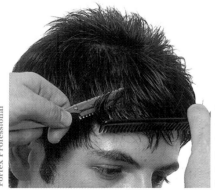

Forfex Professional

(c) Step 4

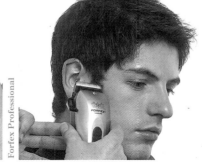

Forfex Professional

(d) Step 6

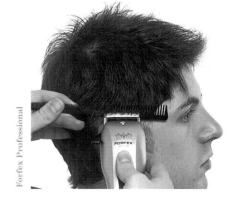

Forfex Professional

(e) Step 8

(f) Step 8

(g) Finished look

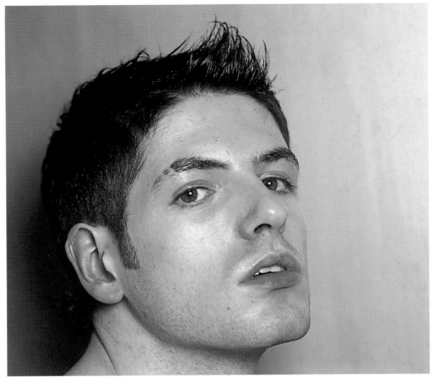

Forfex Professional

Andrea 2 – a shorter highly textured look

1 With the hair wet, comb it back and razor-cut to reduce weight through the front section.

2 Continue this through to the crown area.

3 Move to one side and reduce the length using clippers-over-comb.

4 Increase the length towards the back by increasing the angle of the comb out from the cutting line created at the side. Make sure that the cut blends through without an obvious step in length.

5 Repeat steps 3 and 4 on the other side.

6 Check that the sideburns are level (see tip on page 183) and cut them to the required length and shape.

7 Leave the hair longer in the nape and to the natural hairline at the sides of the neck, but remove unwanted hair outside this outline.

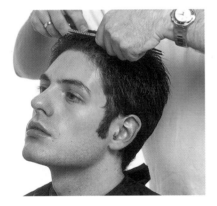

(a) Step 1

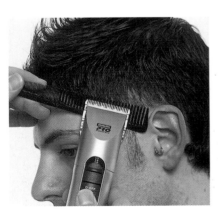

(b) Step 3

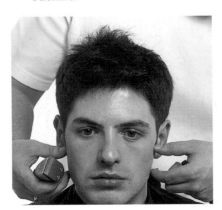

(c) Step 6

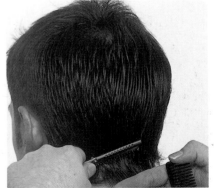

(d) Step 8

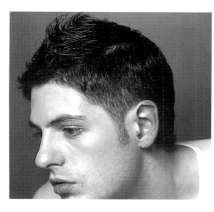

(e) Step 11

(f) Finished look

8 Make sure that the hair is wet at the back and use a razor-tapering technique towards the nape to reduce weight and create texture. Remove small strands of hair around the bottom to break up the outline.

9 One eyebrow can be channelled to create notches for added detail, if required.

10 Shave the areas outside the haircut outlines, if required (see Chapter 11).

11 Blow dry into shape and finish the look with wax or gel to add definition.

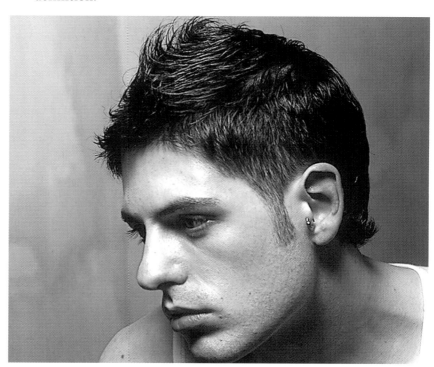

Marcus

1 With the hair wet and combed back, take a section at the front in the centre panel and razor-cut this to length. Take other sections and continue razor-cutting going back along the centre panel towards the crown.

2 Move to the adjacent panel of hair and repeat the process making sure that the panels are connected.

3 Keep working around the top of the head razor-cutting the hair to the length determined by the chosen haircut shape.

4 Move to the side and create movement and texture by razor-cutting the panels down using just the toe of the razor. Take extra care when working against the head if using a razor without a guard fitted.

5 Dress the hair into place to judge how the shape and form is progressing. Razor cut from the sides up into the middle panel of the top to create shorter areas that will break up the movement and support the form being created.

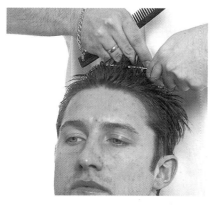

(a) Step 1

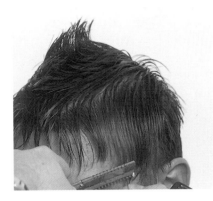

(b) Step 5

6 Remove small strands of hair around the front to break up the outline.

7 Repeat steps 6–8 on the other side and check that the shape is developing symmetrically.

8 Move to one side of the head. Note the required length for any sideburns that may be present, ensure they are level (see tip on page 183) and cut them to shape. Outline the sideburn and around the ears then down the sides of the nape with the tips of your scissors or with the clippers.

9 Using scissors-over-comb, cut the sides around the ear to the correct length and continue around the back to the centre of the head.

10 Repeat this on the other side of the head making sure that the hair blends together where the two sides meet.

11 Create a soft, natural neckline shape by razor-tapering individual strands of hair.

12 Shave the areas outside the haircut outlines, if required (see Chapter 11).

13 Blow dry into shape and finish with wax to add definition.

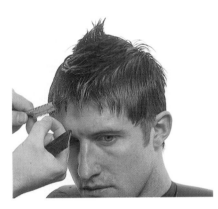

(c) Step 6

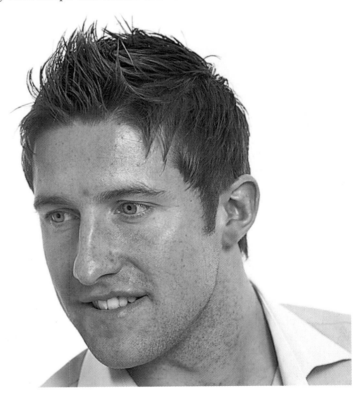

(f) Finished look

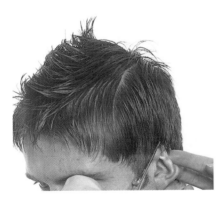

(d) Step 8

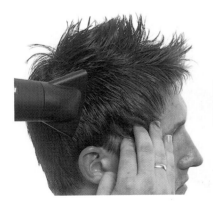

(e) Step 13

Tip

Remember, when determining the correct height for the neckline you should consider the length of the neck, the position of the ears, the head shape and the length of the hair. If the neckline is too low on a short neck it will make the neck appear shorter, whilst if it is too short on a long neck it will make the neck appear longer.

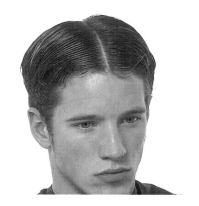

(a) Before cutting

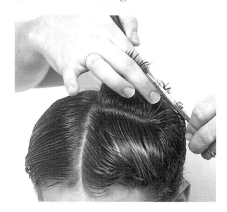

(b) Step 2

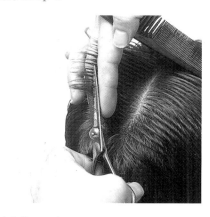

(c) Step 4

Steve H – 'The Pyramid' (colour used to emphasise the cut)

1 First create the basic shape of the pyramid. With the hair wet, section the hair in two by making a parting from the crown to the front. Make a second parting from ear to ear across the top of the head. Take a section parallel to this parting at the crown and hold it at 90° to the head then cut it to length using the scissors-over-fingers technique. Make sure you cut the section at 45° with the highest point in the middle of the head and the lowest at the length required at the sides.

2 Take a section down the centre of the head and cut this at 45° with the longest point at the crown and shortest at the front.

3 Take a section parallel to section 1 and cut this to the guidelines created by both the first and central sections.

4 Continue taking sections parallel to this first section and cutting to the guidelines working down the panel to the front hairline.

5 Transfer the guideline down onto the side of the head by taking a vertical section. Continue cutting these sections to the required length. *Note*: The hair length may be graduated to remove weight around the ears by angling the cut across the section, as required.

6 Transfer the guideline through into the back of the head. The hair length here may also be graduated to remove weight in the nape by angling the cut across the section, as required.

7 Move to the other side and repeat steps 3–6, making sure all panels are connected.

8 Razor-cut the front hairline to add texture and definition.

9 Point cut the top to break up the solid form and enhance movement.

10 Use scissors-over-comb to graduate the bottom of the back and sides, and then outline the sideburns, around the ears and down the sides of the nape with the tips of your scissors.

11 Cut the neckline to the shape required by the look and remove the unwanted hair from outside the outlines.

12 Freehand razor-cutting, using just the toe of the razor is used to create more texture through the sides.

13 Shave the areas outside the haircut outlines, if required (see Chapter 11).

14 The shape is blow dried and finished with gel or wax to add definition.

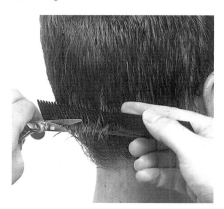

(d) Step 6

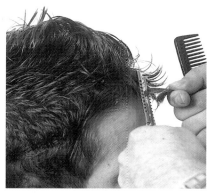

(e) Step 8

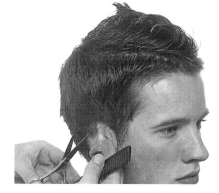

(f) Step 10

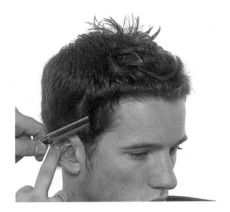

(g) Step 12

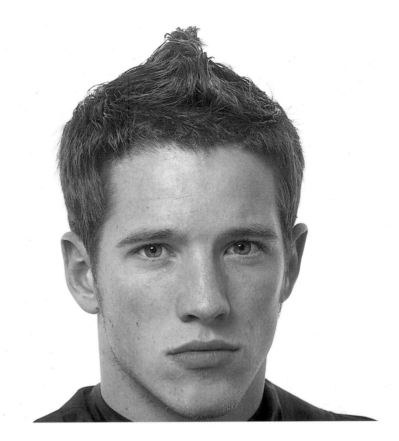

(h) Finished look

Jason – a highly textured look with freehand channelling

1 The hair is point cut and razor-cut through the top to create a disconnected shape with a 40° incline up to the central panel. (Colour can then be applied using techniques, such as flying colours, stippling or polishing – see Chapter 7, 'Colouring men's hair' for more ideas).

2 The hair is then roughly dried into shape.

3 Working with the hair growth pattern at the front, clippers-over-comb is used to create a shorter area between the side and opposite front hairline. This area can be blended into the top or left for a more radical effect.

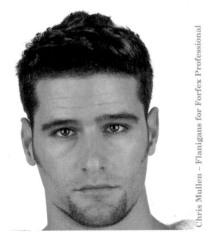

Chris Mullen – Flanigans for Forfex Professional

(a) Before cutting

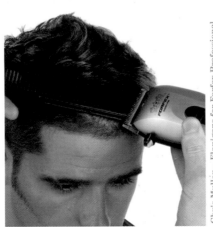

Chris Mullen – Flanigans for Forfex Professional

(b) Step 3

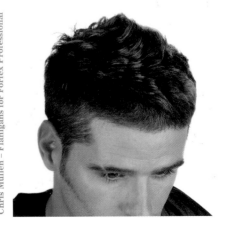

Chris Mullen – Flanigans for Forfex Professional

(c) Step 3

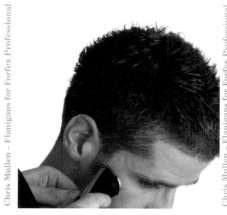

(d) Step 4

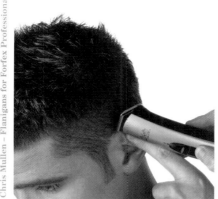

(e) Step 5

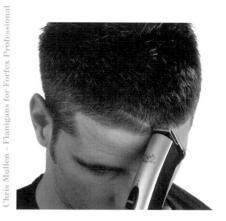

(f) Step 6

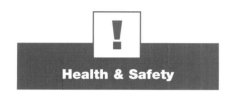

Health & Safety

Remove excess hair cuttings from the client's face and neck at regular intervals to ensure he is comfortable.

4 Continue clippers-over-comb around the back and sides, blending the hair into the shorter area and into the top on the opposite side.

5 Cut the sideburns to the correct length and shape then outline around the ears, sides of the neck and create the neckline. This is probably best tapered.

6 Using a fine blade trimmer, channel a line into the front hairline to create a strong design feature.

7 Shave the areas outside the haircut outlines, if required (see Chapter 11).

8 Finish with wax or gel to add definition and enhance movement.

(g) The finished look

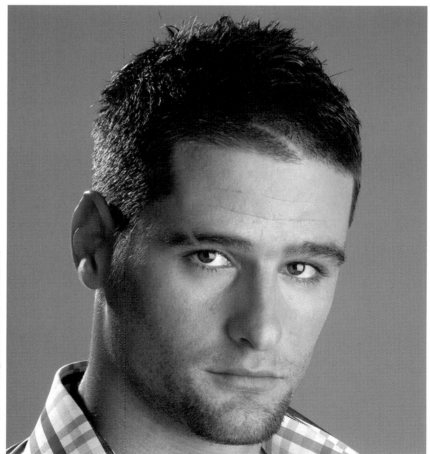

Steve – a skin fade

1   The hair is cut at the back and sides using the clippers set to the longest setting or with a size 1 blade.

2   Ensure that the clippers are placed flat against the neck, just below the neckline. Using a *smooth continuous movement*, push the clippers slowly up the head, keeping them flat against the scalp until you reach the occipital bone. In a smooth *rocking* movement *pivot* the clippers away from the head to produce the shape required.

3   Move to the adjacent panel of hair and repeat the process as before, making sure the panels are connected. Keep working around the head.

4   Move to one side of the head. Note the required length for any sideburns that may be present, ensure they are level and cut them to shape.

5   The neckline and outline must now be tapered to create a natural effect so that the hair appears to fade. Set the clippers to cut at the shortest setting, or use a size 000 blade and hold them directly against the scalp. Pivoting the clippers away in a smooth rocking movement blends and fades the neckline.

6   At the centre panel of hair at the back of the head blend the hair where the top of the taper meets the hair on the top of the head. Move across the head working on small sections and ensure that each panel is connected to blend the two areas together to create an even, continuous effect without any lines.

7   Move across the head following the direction of hair growth and ensure that each panel of hair is connected.

8   The front hairline is then shaped with the clippers.

9   Channelling with the clippers may now be used to create lines, shapes and designs, if required.

10 Scissors- or clippers-over-comb and freehand cutting techniques are then used to shape the top. Make sure that you use even tension throughout the cut, as hair pulled out further and cut will shrink back and leave a hole later.

11 Shave the areas outside the haircut outlines, if required (see Chapter 11).

12 Finish the look with wax to smooth and define the curl movement.

Finished looks

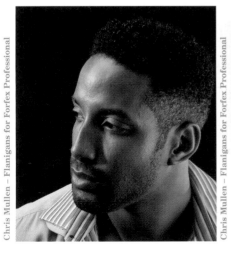

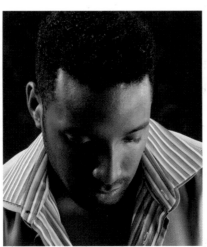

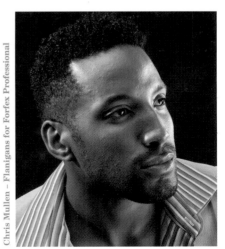

Chris Mullen – Flanigans for Forfex Professional

A flat top

1   Cut the back and sides to about 1 cm or shorter in length using clippers-over-comb or scissors-over-comb techniques. Avoid tapering the bottom of the sides too much. The shape created should appear square and symmetrical when viewed in the mirror. Be careful not to cut into the hair on top of the head at this stage.

2   Move to one side of the head. Note the required length for any sideburns, ensure they are level and cut them to the correct length and shape.

3   The neckline and edge of the outline must now be gently tapered to create a natural look.

4   Wet the top of the hair then dry it straight back into a rough flat top shape. You may need to reduce the overall length of the top first if it is longer than about 5 cm.

5   Start at the crown and use scissors-over-comb or clippers-over-comb techniques to blend the crown area into the hair at the back of the head. This shape can be rounded, as the squared corner shape should begin from the area above the back of the ears.

6   Cut the hair in the central panel to the same length working forwards from the crown. This is the shortest area on top, as the hair length will need to increase to retain the flat shape where the head slopes down towards the sides and front. At the front make sure that your comb stays horizontal – do not let it turn to 90° to follow the shape of the head where it slopes down.

7   Move to the adjacent panel at one side and cut the hair straight across and away from the central guideline in the crown area. Again, here too you must keep the comb horizontal and not let it turn to 90°. The shape you are trying to create is a squared corner. Continue this process along the panel until the head slopes away near the front when you cut to the front guideline. Repeat this on the other side.

8   Take a vertical section at one side above the back of the ear and cut the hair straight up, ensuring that the squared corner shape is retained. Continue this around each side until the squared shape is achieved.

9   You may need to re-wet and blow dry the hair into the flat top shape again before final cutting to make sure all the hairs are lying in their correct positions.

10 Using the previous techniques and freehand cutting, move across the head working on small sections and ensure that each panel is connected to create an even, continuous effect without any lines.

11 Shave the areas outside the haircut outlines, if required (see Chapter 11, 'Shaving').

12 Finish the look with a little wax or hairspray, if required.

Tip

The position of the head is critical when cutting a flat top. If the head is sloping when it is cut, the flat top is likely to slope too! Try to ensure that the client retains his head in a position as though he is looking straight forward whilst walking down a street.

Tip

Flat tops can be cut at many different lengths – you simply adjust the length of the sides and crown area and cut the top to suit.

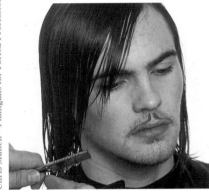

(a) **Before cutting**

A longer look

Jordan – razor-tapering and texturising

1 With the hair wet, take a section at the front and hold it roughly in the shape required. Using a razor-tapering technique cut the hair to the required length around the perimeter of the shape.
2 Continue this process around the side and into the back.
3 Repeat steps 1–2 on the other side.
4 Ensure that the length is even where the two sides meet at the back.
5 Move to the front and create texture by removing strands of hair with just the toe of the razor.
6 Take a section straight out from the crown and hold it at 90°. Reduce the weight towards the perimeter.
7 Take further sections in the adjacent panels, bring the hair to the same position and cut as before. Repeat on the other side.
8 Texturise the outline around the front to break up the solid form and create more movement.
9 Remove any unwanted hair growing on the neck outside the outline.
10 Blow dry into shape and finish with gel or wax to add definition.

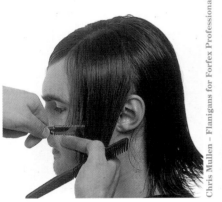

(b) **Step 1**

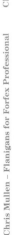

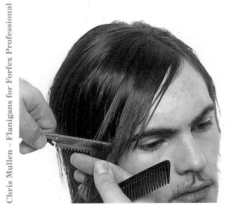

(c) **Step 3**

(d) **Step 4**

(e) **Step 5**

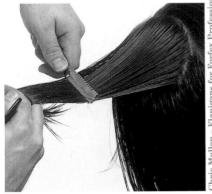

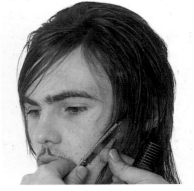

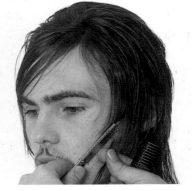

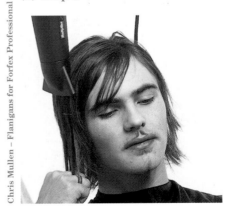

(f) **Step 6**

(g) **Step 8**

(h) **Step 10**

(i) Finished look

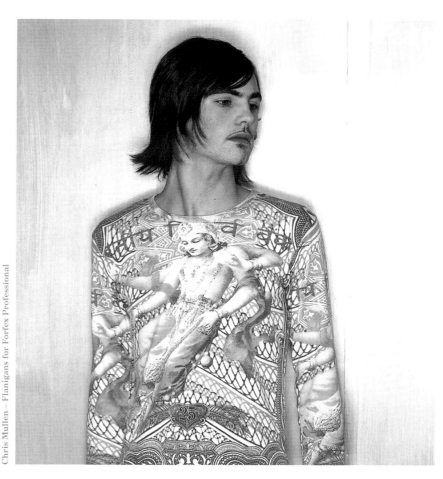

Chris Mullen – Flanigans for Forfex Professional

Health and safety

It is important to consider health and safety when cutting hair because of the risks associated with using electricity and the risk of cutting the skin. Here are some important health and safety factors that you must consider when providing hair-cutting services:

- If the client has any cuts or abrasions on his head, or you suspect that an infection or infestation is present the haircut must not be carried out.
- Pay special attention to hygiene when cutting hair because of the risk of cross-infection through open cuts.
- Open and safety razors have very sharp blades and must always be handled and used with great care.
- Always close the handle to protect the blade of an open razor when it is not being used or when it is being carried.
- *Never* place razors or scissors or other cutting tools in pockets.
- A fixed-blade razor must always be *sterilised* before each use.

- A new blade must always be used for each new client when using a detachable blade open razor.
- Used razor blades, called sharps, must be disposed of correctly in accordance with your salon policy. Soiled disposable materials should be placed in sealed plastic bags for removal.
- Electrical equipment must always be handled and used with care in accordance with the manufacturer's instructions.
- *Never* use or place electric clippers or other electrical equipment near water.
- *Do not* go near electrical equipment that is lying in water – isolate the mains power first.
- Visually check that electrical equipment is safe to use before commencing work – check that the cable has not frayed or been pulled and that the plug is not loose.
- Pay attention to the position of cables when using and storing electrical equipment.
- *Never* overload sockets by plugging too many items of electrical equipment into the same socket.
- Follow the manufacturer's instructions for the care of your scissors and clippers – ensure that you clean and lubricate the blades regularly to avoid damage.
- Only use clean tools and equipment – use alcoholic wipes and sprays to keep clippers clean and disinfected between each client.
- If the client's skin is cut whilst you are cutting his hair stay calm and explain what has happened. Follow your salon's first-aid and accident procedures. Here is an example of what you should do. Give the client a clean dressing and ask him to apply it against the cut until the bleeding stops. A new dressing or plaster may then be applied. Do not touch the cut yourself. Any soiled gowns or towels must be sealed in a plastic bag and laundered at a high temperature, as soon as possible. If the cut is more serious seek medical attention as soon as possible.
- If you cut your own skin whilst you are cutting the client's hair stay calm and explain what has happened. Follow your salon's first-aid and accident procedures. Here is an example of what you should do. Excuse yourself from the client and rinse the cut under cold running water to remove any hairs. Apply a clean dressing against the cut until the bleeding stops. A new dressing or plaster may then be applied. Place any soiled gowns or towels in a plastic bag and seal it. Launder these at a high temperature, as soon as possible. If the cut is more serious seek medical attention as soon as possible.
- Make sure that you know the whereabouts of your salon's first-aid kit. Keep yourself up to date with your salon's first-aid and accident procedures.
- Electrical equipment must be regularly tested and given a certificate of testing to confirm that it is safe for use. Your salon owner will ensure that this is carried out, as required.

Activities

1 Obtain three hair cuttings over 10 cm in length. Club cut one, cutting straight across; taper cut the second and razor cut the third. Compare how the different techniques affect the distribution of weight and movement in the hair cutting.

2 Whilst creating haircuts, try using different texturising techniques and note the effects they produce. Take photographs of the effects (remember to obtain the client's permission first) and make notes. You can then use these to help you explain the techniques to your junior colleagues.

3 Organise a photo shoot in your barber's shop with other colleagues. Create your best work and use the resulting images to publicise your salon or submit them to magazines for wider coverage of your work. Remember to get permission from your manager first.

Check your knowledge

1 Compare the key differences regarding shape and form when producing advanced men's looks to producing basic men's looks.

2 State how techniques are used differently when undertaking advanced cutting.

3 Why is it important to consider hair type when cutting hair?

4 Why should hair colour be considered when cutting hair?

5 Why are neckline shapes important in men's hairdressing?

6 When might it be appropriate to cut into a natural outline?

7 List three points that should be considered when designing sideburn shapes.

8 What is the alternative name for scissor tapering? Describe its effect.

9 Which cutting technique(s) should be carried out on wet hair and not carried out on dry hair?

10 When might razoring be used in haircutting?

11 Describe two texturising techniques.

12 Describe how channelling can be used to emphasise a haircut.

13 Describe a skin fade haircut.

14 Describe how to maintain high standards of hygiene for using electric clippers.

15 What actions should you take if you were to cut your client whilst cutting his hair?

Shaving

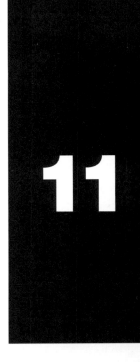

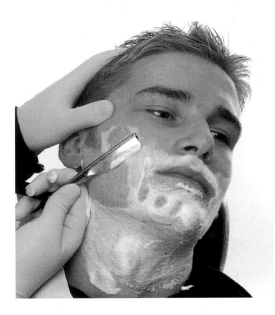

11

Learning objectives

At one time shaving was one of the barber's most popular services, but the introduction of the safety razor and the electric shaver have led to its decline. More recently there has been renewed interest in shaving as a service, particularly in city centre salons that offer a full range of services to the busy professional or traveller.

This chapter looks at the techniques used for shaving and covers the following topics:

- **the decline of shaving in the barber's shop**
- **shaving in the barber's shop today**
- **wet and dry shaving methods**
- **consultation prior to shaving**
- **preparation for shaving**
- **shaving materials – products, tools and equipment**
- **preparing razors for use – including setting and stropping fixed-blade razors**
- **beard preparation – applying hot towels and lather**
- **shaving techniques**
- **a shaving procedure**
- **finishing the shave**
- **common shaving problems**
- **health and safety**

The professional shave

The decline of shaving in the barber's shop

For over 2000 years men have visited the barber's shop regularly for shaving. Indeed, until just a few decades ago many men would visit the barber's shop *daily* for their shave.

At that time shaving was performed with an open, fixed-blade razor, commonly known as a cut-throat razor, which needed regular care to keep it in good working order. Shaving oneself with this type of razor was difficult, time-consuming and often uncomfortable. A shave in the barber's shop, however, was pleasant and relaxing: the barber would perform a face massage, or facial, as part of the service.

The introduction of the safety razor in about 1905 and the introduction of electric shavers in the 1930s made shaving at home much easier. More and more men started shaving themselves and the 'self-shaver' became a feature of modern society. Demand for the 'professional shave' declined further in the 1970s when disposable razors were introduced and the barber's art of shaving was in real danger of being lost.

Shaving in the barber's shop today

The 'self-shaver' is not a completely new phenomenon: self-shavers have existed for hundreds of years. It is the *number* of self-shavers that has had the greatest impact on shaving as a barber's shop service.

Today most men choose to shave because it suits their personal image, or their business or hygiene requirements; shaving is an important part of their personal daily grooming routine. The barber cannot hope to change this, but he can design his services to match his client's shaving routine and experiences. Many men welcome professional advice and information on shaving, particularly if these can help them overcome common shaving problems. Shaving products, equipment and skin-care products are also in constant demand by the self-shaver. Men must still get their hair cut and for this most visit the salon. Today the opportunities clearly exist for the barber to introduce his clients to shaving services.

Here are some ideas to consider if you are interested in providing shaving services:

- Offer shaving (and face massage) services for special occasions such as weddings.
- Offer shampooing, blow-drying and shaving services to travellers and other busy men.
- Offer instruction on how to shave effectively.

- Provide advice on shaving problems. For example, many men have difficulty shaving their sideburns level – they use their ears to judge the balance, but on most people the ears are not level. You can show them how to do this correctly. You can also discuss ways of avoiding razor burn, and so on.
- Provide advice on products. It will help if you also stock these products!

Shaving

The purpose of shaving is to remove the visible part of the hair and leave the skin smooth to touch. This is achieved by means of a razor or some other tool that cuts the hair close to the skin. A good shave is achieved without irritating the skin. Both men and women regularly practise shaving but here we will only consider its use on men within the salon.

The professional shave is used to remove unwanted hair from the face and neck. It may be used to outline moustaches, beards, sideburns and necklines or to remove all visible beard hair.

Wet and dry shaving methods

A shave may be achieved by either wet or dry methods.

Dry shaving

Dry shaving uses an electric shaver, which may be powered by disposable or rechargeable batteries, or by mains electricity.

There are many different types of electric shaver, but typically they all consist of a number of sharp cutting blades that move rapidly to cut the hair when power is applied. The blades move behind a very thin flexible guard, which both protects the skin and positions the hairs for optimum cutting.

Electric shavers are mostly used by the self-shaver, and are particularly suitable for the busy professional or traveller. They are easy to carry and can be used with ease in almost any location, especially if powered by batteries. However, they are less suitable for use in the salon, as they are more difficult to sterilise and do not provide such a close shave.

Wet shaving

Wet shaving is the method of shaving traditionally used in the salon. It is achieved by means of a razor, which can either be an open ('cut-throat') razor or a safety razor.

In wet shaving the area to be shaved is prepared by the application of lather, gel or shaving oil prior to shaving. The hairs are then removed with a razor while they are still wet.

The open razor comprises a very sharp steel blade which is protected by a hinged cover when not in use. Safety razors have a thin guard covering the blade, which both protects the skin and positions the blade and hair for optimum cutting. Several different types of safety razor are available: some are totally disposable, whilst others have a detachable blade that is easily replaced when a new blade is required.

Consultation prior to shaving

Consultation is an essential part of any hairdressing service, and is particularly important when shaving because of the risks associated with the use of razors.

Time must always be given to discussing the client's requirements with him. It is essential that careful consideration be given to each of the following factors before any lather is applied to the face.

- What does the client want? Does he want a close shave?
- Does he have a moustache, a beard or sideburns? If so, does he wish to keep them?
- Look for signs of broken skin, abnormalities on the skin, and any unusual beard growth patterns.
- Is the beard hair coarse or fine?
- Is the beard growth dense or sparse?

There are other factors that affect the way you carry out the shave. The following are the most important:

- hair growth patterns
- hair texture
- density of the beard
- the facial features

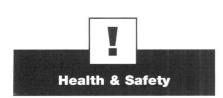

Health & Safety

A thorough consultation will ensure that you identify any adverse conditions of the hair or skin that may be present. It is particularly important to establish whether a suspected infection or infestation is present: this would prevent you from carrying out the shave. (This area is covered more fully in Chapter 2, 'Client care for men'.)

Tip

The 'first time over' shave should always be carried out *following* the direction of hair growth.

Hair growth patterns

Hair growth patterns are the ways in which individual hairs or a section of the beard may grow in a particular direction. Hair growth patterns must be identified, and the 'first time over' shave should always be carried out *following* the direction of the hair growth. (Shaving *against* the hair growth at the start of the shave would cause the razor to drag, and would be very uncomfortable for the client.)

If the client requests a close shave, shaving against the direction of growth may be performed during the 'second time over' shave. Care should be taken not to shave the hair *too* close, however, as this would irritate the skin and might cause 'ingrown hairs', particularly on men with curly hair. Ingrown hairs can become infected and may lead to conditions such as impetigo or folliculitis.

Some clients have very strong hair growth patterns in their beard, such as hair whorls. In such cases, shave by following the direction of hair growth around the whorl.

Tip

Ask your client whether there are any areas he finds difficult to shave. Each client is usually an expert when it comes to identifying problem areas on his own face!

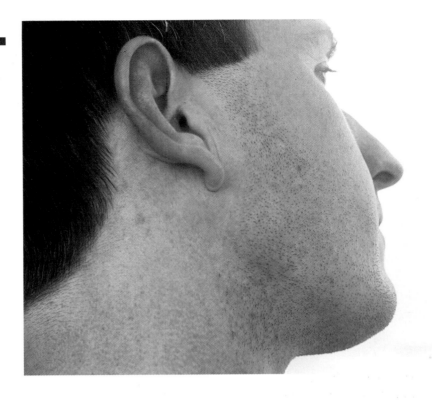

Tip

Very dense and coarse beards should be steamed with a hot towel and well lathered before shaving: the steam and lather help to soften the beard. The lather should be massaged into the beard for a few minutes and then reapplied before commencing the shave.

Tip

Facial piercings should be removed, if possible, prior to shaving unless the area around the piercing is affected by keloids. If left in place, mark its position in the lather and make the razor stoke away from the piercing.

Texture

As with all hair, the texture of hair in a beard can be fine, medium or coarse. Fine hair is easy to shave, as it creates little resistance to the razor. Coarse hair can be very difficult to shave and requires much more lather and massaging to soften the beard before shaving. Young men usually have fine facial hair, but as men get older their facial hair often becomes much coarser.

Density

Hair density means the amount of hair that grows in a given area of skin. This is important to consider in shaving as the density of the growth may make it necessary to carry out a 'second time over' shave.

Young men often have sparse facial hair growth, but this becomes denser as they get older. Some men have very dense beard growth, often called 'blue beards' as the density of growth gives the skin a blue tinge which remains even after shaving. Men with very dense beards may have to shave twice a day to keep a clean-shaven appearance. Not surprisingly, they may decide to stop shaving and grow beards.

Facial features

To prevent damage to the skin it is important to identify and consider the client's facial features. Careful note should be made of the following:

- the mouth
- the width of the top lip
- the nose
- the shape of the jaw and chin
- any unusual features, such as moles, dimples, scarring or piercings

Preparation for shaving

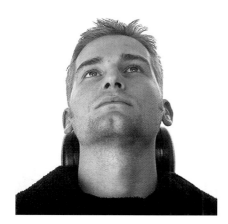

The prepared client

1. Carry out your consultation with the client. Look for signs of broken skin, abnormalities on the skin, and unusual beard growth patterns.
2. Agree with your client the methods of shaving that you will use.
3. Before you begin work, gather together all the materials, products, tools and equipment you will require.
4. Position the client in a reclining chair with support for his head. Use a clean paper towel over the headrest.
5. Gown the client and place a clean towel across his chest, tucked in at the neck. Place a clean paper towel over the towel and across his shoulder (from the client's neck towards your body).
6. Your hands and nails should be clean: let your client see that you have washed them. Make sure that the razor has been prepared correctly. Show your client that you have sterilised the razor or that you are fitting a new blade – make it clear that you use high standards of hygiene in your work.

Tip

After applying lather, mark the position of any moles, dimples, scarring or piercings by removing the lather from these areas with a tissue. Always make the razor stroke moving *away* from the mole, dimple, scar or piercing or you might cut the skin and/or damage the razor!

Shaving materials, products, tools and equipment

Materials

Required materials include the following. First, you will need hot and cool towels. Unless they are specially supplied pre-packed for shaving, these should be sterilised. You will also need a roll of tissue paper, for wiping used lather from the razor.

In case of any accidents, you must have access to first-aid materials. For small nicks or cuts you will need styptic liquid or powder. You

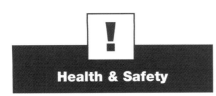

Health & Safety

Always wear gloves, to avoid the risk of cross-infection. They should be tight-fitting so that you can use the razor and tension the skin effectively during the shave. Try to use gloves that are free from latex to avoid problems with clients who have allergies to latex.

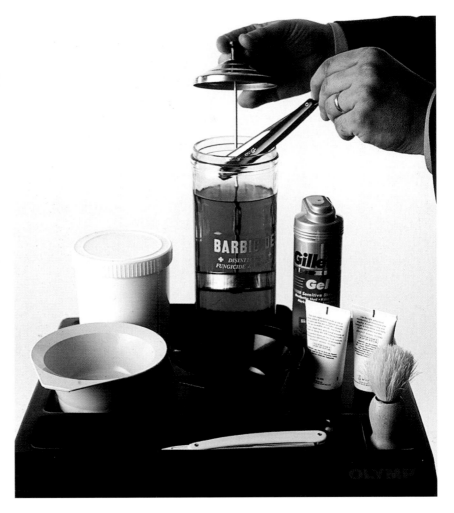

Barbicide

may use a styptic pencil, but only once – you must use a fresh one for each new client.

To avoid the risk of cross-infection, you should wear gloves.

Products

To carry out the shave you will need shaving soaps, foam or gel, for lathering the face, or shaving oil, to ensure that the face is adequately lubricated.

To finish you may need products such as aftershave lotions, aftershave balms, moisturisers and talcum powder.

Tools

Open razors

Open razors are usually used in barbering. They have either a fixed blade, which must be sharpened or set, or a detachable blade, which is disposable. Open razors, also known as 'cut-throat' razors, have a hinged handle that closes to protect the blade when not in use.

- Open razors have very sharp blades: they must always be treated with care and respect. Keep the handle closed to cover the blade when not in use, and especially when carrying or passing the razor. Never place a razor in your pocket. Always keep razors out of the reach of children.

- When passing an open razor, the handle must always be closed. In addition, wrap your hand around it to prevent it from opening accidentally. Pass the razor with the tang facing away from you and towards the other person.

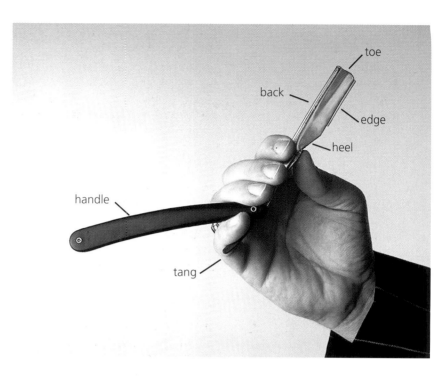

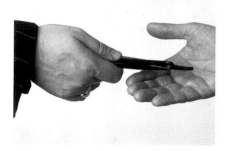

(a) Correct: tang facing away

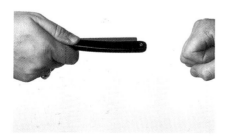

(b) Incorrect

Fixed-blade razors

Fixed-blade razors can be either 'hollow-ground' or 'solid-ground'. They were the preferred choice of traditional barbers for many years, but are more difficult to use commercially because they have to be sterilised before use on each client.

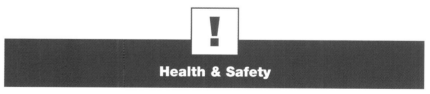

- A different fixed-blade razor should be kept for each client's personal use: the razor should be used on no one else. Fixed-blade razors must *always* be effectively sterilised before use.

- Before using a fixed-blade razor for shaving, check your local by-laws. In many areas the use of fixed-blade razors is prohibited. (Your local council will be able to help you.)

Note: It is good practice to use disposable blade open razors for professional shaving services.

📎 Tip

Fully disposable razors are sometimes used in the salon, but they are usually designed for home use, and are not as effective for the professional shave.

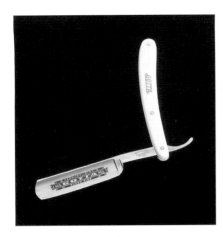

A hollow-ground razor

Hollow-ground razors may be of either German or English origin. They have a concave appearance when viewed end-on, and are made of hardened steel. The steel undergoes a special heat treatment called tempering, which gives the razor the correct degree of hardness to produce a good cutting edge. Hollow-ground razors are usually 'hard-tempered', which makes them more difficult to sharpen (set), but the sharp edge lasts longer. Hollow-ground razors are light and have a particular feel that is much preferred by most barbers, especially when carrying out shaving. They are less suitable for cutting hair.

Solid-ground or French razors have a wedge-shaped blade that is much heavier and more rigid than the hollow-ground razor. They too are made of hardened steel and are usually 'soft-tempered', which makes them easier to sharpen, but the sharp edge does not last as long. Due to their greater weight and rigidity they are suitable for cutting hair, but they are difficult to use when shaving.

Detachable-blade razors

Detachable-blade razors are the preferred choice for professional shaving today because they are more hygienic than fixed-blade razors. They are designed to be very similar to a hollow-ground razor but they have disposable blades, which are easily replaced. Some detachable blade razors come with special dispensers that store new blades and help attach them without their being handled.

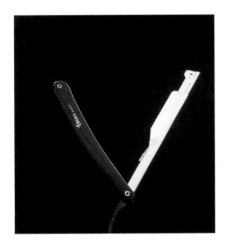

A detachable-blade razor

The hair shaper is a type of detachable-blade razor that has a removable guard over the blade. These are not really suitable for shaving as the toe of the blade forms a point which can easily cut the skin when in use. However, they are good for haircutting because the guard can be left in place to help control the amount of hair being removed.

Equipment

An adjustable chair

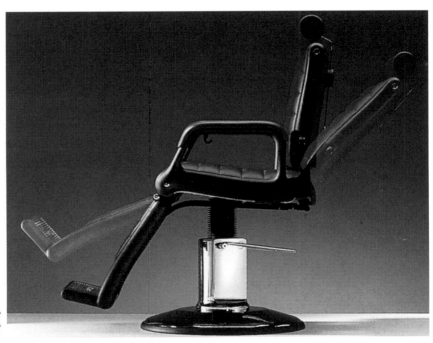

Olymp

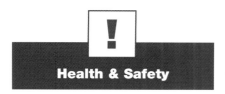

Health & Safety

Remember to lock the chair before the client sits down and again whilst carrying out the shave so that it does not swivel and cause accidents.

The client should be seated in an adjustable chair, which can be positioned so that the client can recline comfortably while he is being shaved. It should have a headrest, and the height of the chair should be adjusted so that you do not have to bend uncomfortably.

A hone and strop will be required if you intend using fixed-blade razors. You may also need a shaving brush and a shaving mug or bowl, particularly if you intend to use shaving soaps. The shaving brush and mug must be cleaned thoroughly in disinfectant and sterilised between clients. This is often difficult to do commercially, and it is easier to keep a personal brush and sometimes a new mug for each client.

Preparing razors for use

Setting fixed-blade razors

Hollow-ground and solid-ground razors have to be sharpened or set to keep them in good working order. The process of setting a razor is commonly called honing, as the razor is sharpened on a hone.

Honing is a process that requires a great deal of skill to ensure that the edge of the razor is set correctly. The edge of a razor has a number of very fine teeth cut into it that have a saw-like appearance if viewed under a microscope. The teeth make the razor sharp. The process of honing sets new teeth into the edge of the razor and realigns any older teeth that remain.

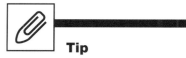

Health & Safety

Take great care when testing the edge of the razor using the thumbnail method. Ensure you apply no pressure or the razor will easily cut in to the nail.

The razor edge may easily be damaged or over-honed during honing so the razor should be tested frequently to determine the degree of sharpness. The simplest way to test the razor's edge is to place it *very carefully* and *lightly* on a moistened thumbnail. Slowly draw the nail along a little from the heel to the toe of the razor: if the razor tugs the nail with a smooth and steady grip, the edge is sharp.

Hones

Various types of hones are available for sharpening razors. They usually consist of a rectangular block of abrasive material, which because it is harder than steel cuts the edge of the razor. Most barbers have a preferred choice of hone, acquired through years of experience.

Hones can be divided into three main groups, depending on what they are made of: natural, synthetic, and combination.

Natural hones come from naturally occurring rock formations. They usually have to be lubricated with water or lather before use, and have a slow cutting action that produces a very fine and long-lasting edge. Water hones, which come from Germany, and Belgian hones are two popular varieties of natural hone.

Tip

Great care should be taken when using a synthetic hone to avoid over-honing the razor edge.

Synthetic hones are man-made and can be used either wet or dry. Their cutting action is much faster than that of natural hones and they can produce a good cutting edge in less time. It is particularly important to test the razor edge regularly when using a synthetic hone, as it is very easy to over-hone a razor with a hone that cuts quickly! A carborundum hone is a popular type of synthetic hone.

Combination hones are the preferred choice of many barbers. They have two working sides: one side is a natural hone, the other a synthetic hone. The synthetic side is used to quickly cut a new edge on the razor. The natural side is then used to produce a very fine and long-lasting finished edge.

The method of setting hollow-ground razors

1 Lubricate the hone with water, lather or oil, as recommended by the manufacturer.
2 Place the razor flat on the hone, with the edge facing towards the middle (a).
3 Using light pressure, slide the blade across the hone, moving diagonally from the heel to toe (b).
4 Rotate the razor between the thumb and forefinger whilst keeping the back of the razor on the hone – keep rotating until the razor edge is pointing straight up.
5 Using no pressure push the razor up the hone away from your body until the heel is level with the bottom edge of the hone (c).
6 Continue rotating the razor, as before, to make the blade lie flat with its edge again facing the middle of the hone (d).
7 Slide the blade back across the hone, moving diagonally from heel to toe (e, f).

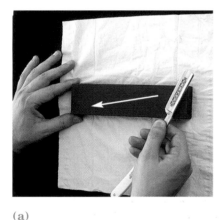

(a)

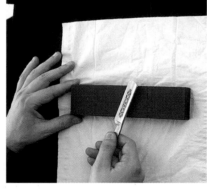

(b)

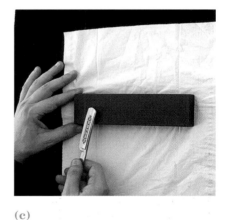

(c)

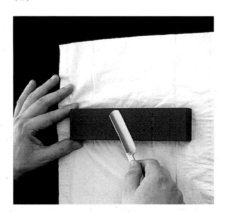

(d)

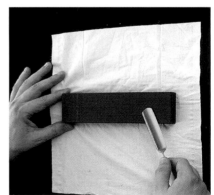

(e)

(f)

8   Repeat these movements several times.

9   Every few strokes of the hone, test the development of the edge by gently and carefully placing the razor edge on a moistened thumbnail. Slowly draw the nail along a little from the heel to the toe of the razor: if the razor tugs the nail with a smooth and steady grip the edge is sharp.

Stropping fixed-blade razors

The razor strop is used to give the razor a smooth 'whetted' edge. Stropping a razor does not cut into the steel, as honing does; instead, it cleans or polishes the edge, depending on which side of the strop is used. There are two main types of strop available: hanging strops, and French or German strops.

Hanging strops are usually combination strops that consist of canvas on one side and leather on the other. As their name implies, they are designed to hang from a swivel attached to one end (as illustrated below). Hanging strops are mostly used for stropping hollow-ground razors and are preferred by most barbers. French or German strops are usually made of wood and covered, again with canvas on one side and leather on the other. They are mainly used for stropping solid-ground razors and are less common.

A hanging strop

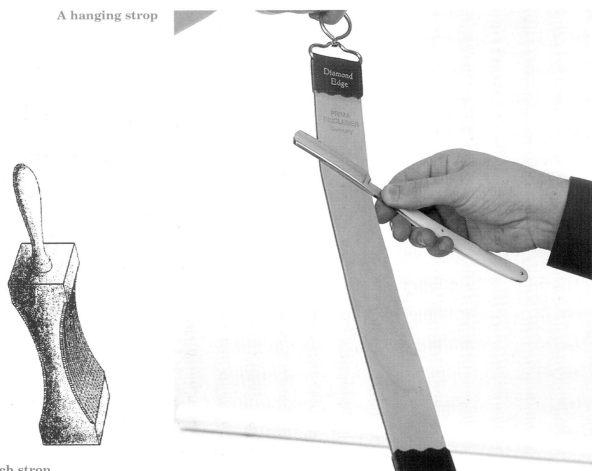

A French strop

Tip

Remember, the canvas side of the strop should be used first, as this cleans the edge of the blade. This must always be followed with the leather side to polish it and produce a smooth whetted edge.

Tip

A lot of practice is required to be able to strop a razor quickly and effectively. It is a good idea to practise with an old razor on an old strop. Make the movements slowly at first – increase the speed only when you become more proficient.

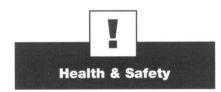

Health & Safety

Always sterilise razors after stropping.

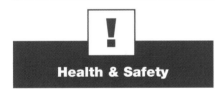

Health & Safety

A new blade must be fitted for each client.

New strops usually have to be 'broken in' before they will work effectively. Breaking in should be carried out following the manufacturer's recommendations. A method frequently used involves rubbing pumice stone across the surface to make the strop smooth. Stiff lather is then rubbed in repeatedly. Finally, and after some time, a smooth bottle or glass is rubbed over the strop until a very smooth surface is achieved.

The *canvas* side of a strop is used to clean the razor's edge and realign the cutting teeth, which become unaligned when the razor is used. The strop's effect is similar to mild honing, so a freshly honed razor should not be stropped using the canvas side. The *leather* side of a strop is made of cowhide, horsehide or imitation leather. Horsehide strops are usually of higher quality and are more expensive. The leather side polishes the edge to create a smooth finish, which is commonly called a whetted edge. This is achieved when all the very fine teeth on the razor edge are clean and aligned in the direction of the shaving stroke.

The method of stropping razors

The action used for stropping is similar to the action used in honing, but the razor is moved with *the back facing the direction of movement*. (Moving the razor with the edge facing the direction of movement would both cut the strop and damage the razor!)

1 Place the razor flat on the strop with the back facing towards the middle (a).

2 Using light pressure, slide the blade across the strop, moving diagonally from the heel to toe (b).

3 Rotate the razor between the thumb and forefinger, keeping the back of the razor on the strop – keep rotating until the razor edge is pointing straight up (c).

4 Using no pressure, push the razor across the strop away from your body until the heel is level with the edge of the strop (d).

5 Continue rotating the razor as before, until the blade lies flat with its back again facing the middle of the strop.

6 Slide the blade back across the strop, moving diagonally from heel to toe (e).

7 Repeat these movements several times.

Tip

Show your client that you have sterilised the fixed-blade razor, or that you are fitting a new blade to a detachable-blade razor. Making it clear that you have high standards of hygiene in your work will give clients confidence.

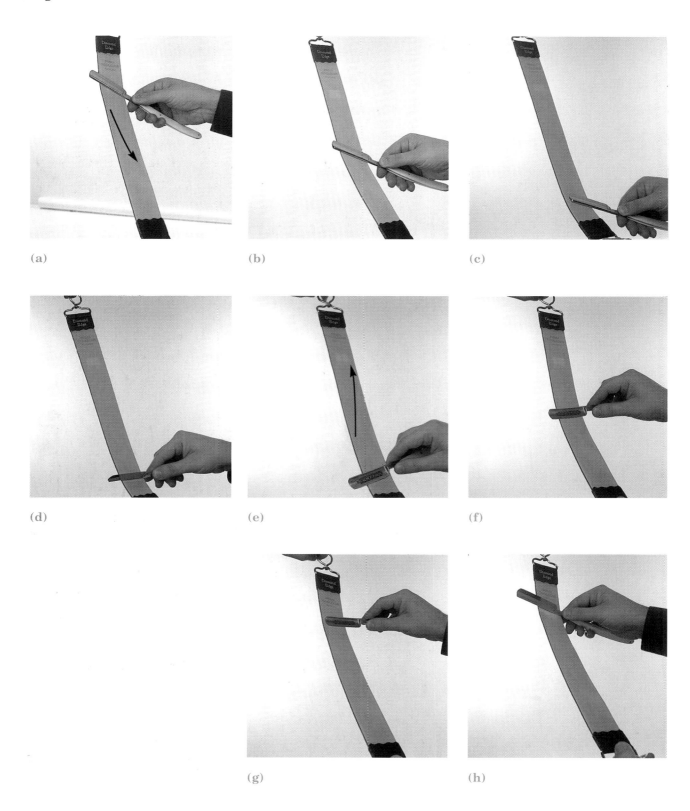

(a)

(b)

(c)

(d)

(e)

(f)

(g)

(h)

Detachable-blade razors

Used blades (known as sharps) must be removed carefully and disposed of in a suitable container (see 'health and safety' on page 224). The razor must then be thoroughly washed in disinfectant.

Preparing the beard

Ensure that the client's face and beard are visibly clean. Long beard growth that is to be removed should be disentangled as necessary, and the excess hair removed with scissors and clippers before starting the shave.

A beard must be softened before shaving is attempted. Softening the beard is achieved through the application of hot towels and lather.

Applying hot towels

Hot towels steam the face and help in these ways:

- they remove dirt
- they soften the hair cuticle
- they lubricate the face, by stimulating the oil-producing glands
- they relax the muscles, making shaving easier
- they relax the client

A rolled-up towel retains heat

You must use *clean* towels. Some barbers use pre-packed towels, which are specially supplied ready-sterilised.

Hot towels are prepared in a steamer or by soaking them in hot water. Wring out the towel until it is nearly dry, then roll it up so that it retains its heat while you carry it to the client.

Unroll the towel and wrap it around the client's face, being careful not to cover the nose, so that the client can breathe. Allow the towel to cool.

The cool towel should be replaced by a second (and if necessary a third) hot towel, which should be left on while you prepare the lather.

When using hot towels, remember the following important points:

- Always use clean towels for each new client.
- Prepare and apply the towels as quickly as possible but be sure to work safely – the quicker you are the more effective they will be.
- Avoid covering the client's nose.
- The towels should by nearly dry when they are applied.
- Remove the last hot towel before it becomes too cold – lather should be applied to a warm face!

Health & Safety

Always test the temperature of the towel on the client's chin before wrapping to ensure that it is not too hot.

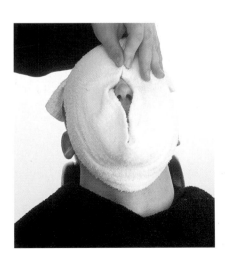

Lathering

Effective lathering is essential to a good shave. Lathering is used:

- to remove dirt
- to soften the hair

- to lift individual hairs so that they stand erect from the skin for cutting
- to lubricate the face so that the razor glides more easily

Traditionally the method used to produce a rich lather was to vigorously work a shaving brush into a bar of shaving soap and a shaving mug containing warm water. 'Working up' a good lather was necessary, as the consistency of the lather was critical to the success of the shave. The lather had to be slightly watery at first to hydrate the skin and stop the lather from drying out too quickly. The stiffness of the lather was then increased to hold the hairs erect and provide adequate lubrication for the razor.

Modern shaving products are designed to produce instant lather. They contain conditioners to help protect the face and to stop the lather from drying out too quickly. Some are in the form of gels and oils which do not produce lather but have the same effect. Shaving soaps are still available for those who wish to use them – they work well but require more preparation – so it is purely a personal choice.

Traditional lather has to be applied with a shaving brush, but modern products can be applied easily without the need for brushes or bowls. The use of the shaving brush does have additional benefits, though: the circular, upward motion used when applying the lather helps to work the lather into the beard and make the hairs stand erect.

Here are some important points to bear in mind when applying lather:

- The lather should be applied immediately after the last hot towel has been removed.
- The lather should be applied starting under the tip of the chin (a). It is best applied with a lathering brush in an upward, circular motion which rotates in small circles over the face (b, c).

(a)

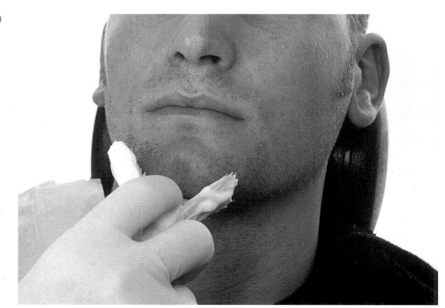

(b)

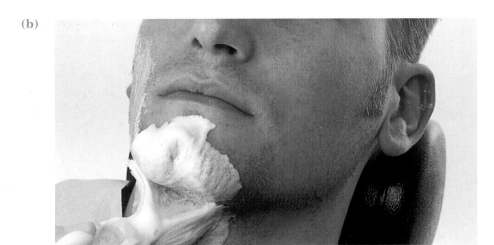

(c)

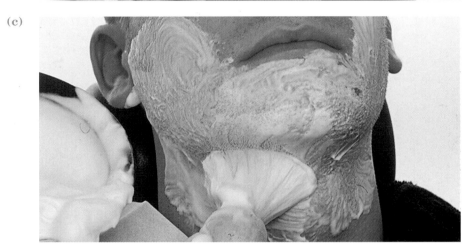

(d)

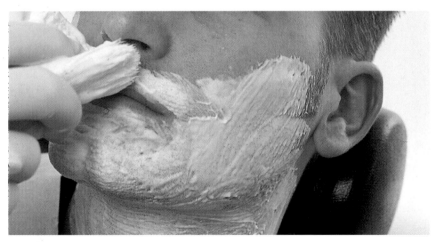

Tip

Before each shaving stroke, make sure that the lather is still creamy and moist. Dry lather will not adequately lubricate the face: this will make the razor pull, causing considerable discomfort to the client. Always apply more lather first, as required.

- The top lip is best lathered with a splayed brush, obtained by placing the index finger in the centre of the bristles (d). This avoids any lather going up the client's nose or into his mouth.

- On dense or coarse beards, the lather should be massaged into the beard for a few minutes with three fingers of either hand, and then reapplied with the brush.

- Do not let the lather run or drip, or dry out before shaving.

Shaving techniques

Tip

Try to carry out your first shave on a fine or sparse beard – this will create less resistance to the razor, be easier to achieve, and will therefore help build your confidence.

Avoid shaving older men during your first shaves, as older skin tends to be more 'wrinkly' and less elastic. Because it usually requires more tension to make it smooth, older skin is more difficult to shave.

The shaving procedure should be systematic. To be effective you require good co-ordination of both hands and the correct use of techniques. These are skills that take a lot of practice to develop.

You must be able to perform the techniques adequately *before* you try shaving anyone. A good way to practise is by shaving a lathered balloon with an old razor. (Ask someone to hold the balloon firmly for you while you do this.) If you burst the balloon, you were using too much pressure or holding the razor incorrectly. Alternatively, you could remove the blade from a detachable blade open razor and practice with this on a model. *Make doubly sure you have removed the blade before commencing.*

This method of practising is only of use in developing 'the feel' of the razor against a delicate surface. Eventually you must make your first shaving stroke for real! You must be supervised when you do this. Work slowly and carefully, and try to remain relaxed and supple.

Holding the razor

Hold the razor in either your right or left hand, as best suits you. This hand is called your shaving hand. The correct way of holding the razor for a right-handed person is illustrated below. For a left-handed person the razor is simply reversed.

Tensioning the skin

Your other hand is used to tension the skin. This is called your tensioning hand. You must keep the fingers of this hand dry, to prevent them from slipping on the face.

The tensioning hand should be placed at the back of the razor so that you can stretch the skin under the razor before carrying out each stroke.

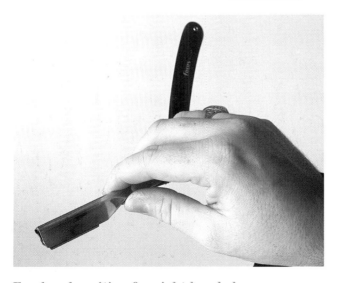

Forehand position for right-handed person

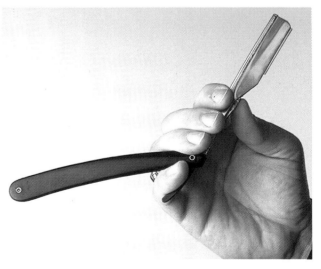

Backhand position for a right-handed person

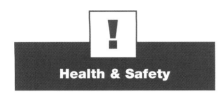

Health & Safety

If you use shaving soap blocks and shaving brushes, you must keep a separate set for each client.

Shaving

The shaving stroke is performed with a single gliding movement. Try to avoid making short movements unless shaving a small area, as the razor will tend to 'pull' more and shaving will be less effective.

The forehand (sometimes called freehand) stroke is made towards you, and the backhand stroke away from you. Keep the razor at the correct cutting angle, about 40–45°, throughout the stroke. Do not apply too much pressure: the action should be light and free-moving.

Eventually you will develop a 'feel' for the correct angles and pressure to use. This feel or touch is known as the barber's hand, and when acquired it will allow you to make perfect shaves both safely and efficiently.

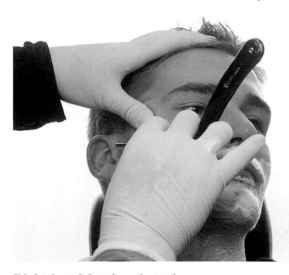

Right-hand forehand stroke

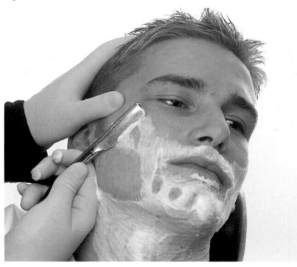

Right-hand backhand stroke

A shaving procedure

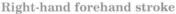

First time over

The shave should start on the nearest side to the barber – a right-handed barber stands on the right side of the client, a left-handed barber on the left side.

The skin must always be stretched taut before carrying out the stroke with the razor, otherwise cuts may occur and the shave will not be very close. After making sure they are level, mark the position of the sideburns by drawing your finger across the lather.

On the first-time-over shave, shaving follows the direction of beard growth in the pattern of ten strokes illustrated in the photographs on the following page. After each stroke, wipe the razor clean on the bottom of the tissue, then fold the tissue to cover the used lather. Keep wiping the razor this way until about three-quarters of the tissue length has been used, then replace the used tissue with a new one from the roll. Make sure you dispose of the used tissue correctly.

A typical pattern of shaving
strokes

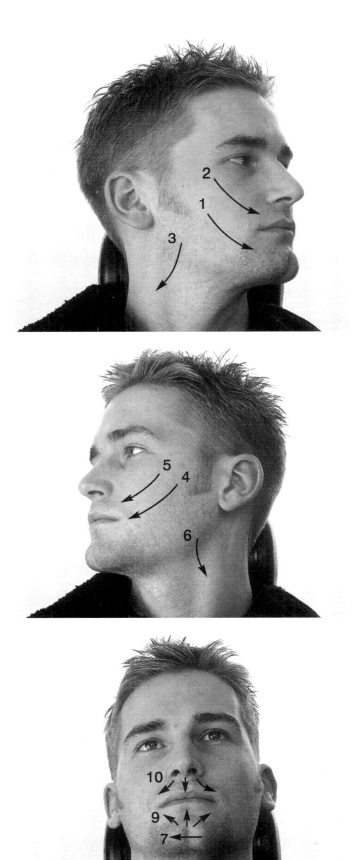

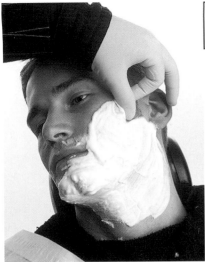

Tip

To ensure that the sideburns are shaved level, place one finger high on each sideburn. Whilst looking in the mirror slide one finger down until the desired length is reached. Slide the other finger down until both fingers are level. Mark the position of both fingers by drawing them across the lather.

Marking the sideburns

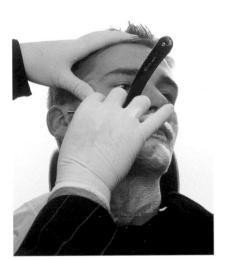

Stroke 1

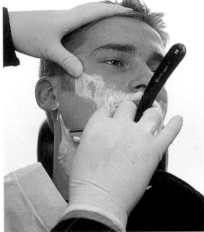

Stroke 1

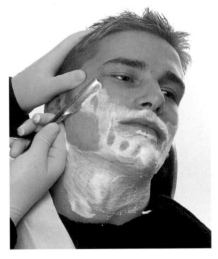

Stroke 2

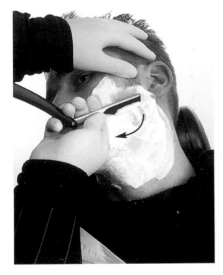

Stroke 4

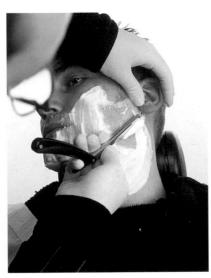

Stroke 4

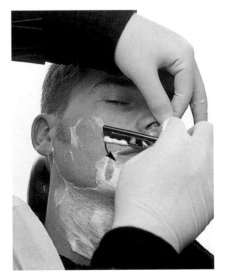

Stroke 10

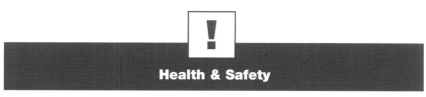

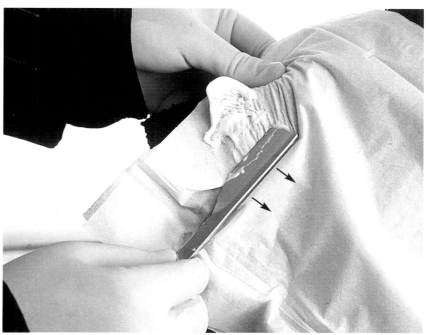

When wiping the razor, keep the blade flat and wipe it away from the edge. Never wipe along the blade or wrap the tissue around the blade as serious cuts would surely occur.

Second time over

This shave is carried out *against* the beard growth, to get a closer shave finish. This is not always required, especially on immature or fine beards.

The second-time-over shave is usually the final shave unless the client has a strong beard growth or a very close shave is required, in which case a sponge shave may be carried out. In the sponge shave a clean, sterilised sponge, which has been dipped in hot water, is slowly drawn across the face, closely followed by the razor. The damp sponge lubricates the face and raises the hairs into the path of the razor for close cutting. The sponge shave produces a very close shave: great care must be taken not to shave the hairs *too* close.

The once-over shave

The once-over shave is the method used by experienced barbers to achieve a good even finish without having to re-lather the face and carry out a second time over. It is achieved by making a few more shaving strokes, as follows.

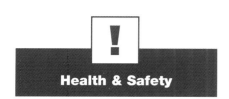

A new sponge must be used for each new client.

Be very careful not to shave the hair too close, as this would irritate the skin and could cause ingrown hairs. This is particularly likely with curly hair.

Once-over shave: shaving
against the hair growth

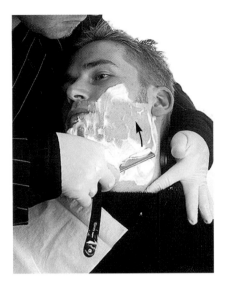

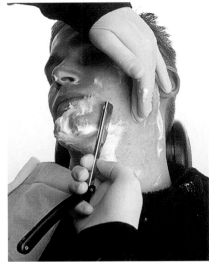

Shaving a beard outline

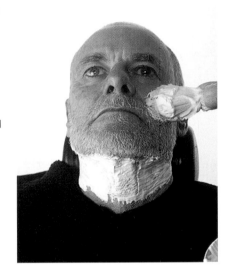

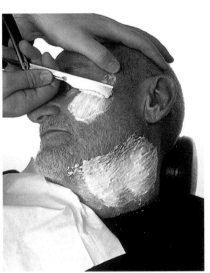

Tip

Extra care should be taken when shaving the outlines of sideburns and moustaches. Make sure that you mark their outline by drawing your finger through the lather before shaving. Men are often very protective of their sideburn or moustache shape, and mistakes will not go unnoticed – especially right under their noses!

- After completing each shaving stroke, feel for remaining hair growth by running the fingers of your tensioning hand gently across the face.
- Where you feel hair growth remaining, gently complete a shaving stroke against the hair growth – being very careful not to shave too close.

The neck shave

The neck shave is often used to prolong the clean appearance outside the outline of a haircut on the neck and behind the ears.

It is performed with the same techniques used when shaving the face. Note the following points.

- The client should be gowned, with the towel placed around the back of the neck.
- If the hair is very fine, the lather may be replaced with a little warm water.

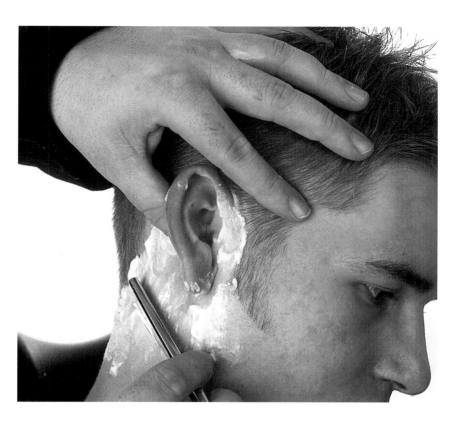

- Stand to the side of the client. If you are right-handed, use a forehand stroke to shave the right side of the neck and a backhand stroke for the left side. If you are left-handed, reverse this.

- When shaving near the ears, protect them by folding them back gently with your tensioning hand.

- Finish the shave by applying a small amount of talcum powder, antiseptic or moisturiser. An aftershave lotion may be applied if the client wishes.

Finishing the shave

When the shave has been completed you may apply hot towels and carry out a face massage if your client requires this. If a face massage is not required, the face should be cleaned with a warm, damp towel or sponge, and then gently patted dry with a clean towel. Some clients enjoy the cooling and soothing effects of a cool towel: this is prepared and used just like a hot towel, but using cool water. Other clients even enjoy the bracing effects of a very cold towel, but you should ask before this is applied.

A small amount of talcum powder or moisturiser may be applied to soothe and smooth the skin. An aftershave lotion or aftershave balm may also be applied, if the client so desires. Aftershave *lotions* have a bracing effect on the skin – they are astringent. Aftershave *balms* are less astringent and are preferred by men who do not care for this bracing effect. Both help to close the pores of the face, reducing the risk of infection.

Tip

Remember to comb and style the client's hair as requested before he leaves the chair.

Tip

If the client is having a face massage after shaving, apply a warm towel when the lather has been removed. The face should be warm and the facial muscles relaxed for face massage.

Common wet shaving problems

The table identifies some common wet shaving problems, possible causes and their remedies.

Problem	Possible cause	Possible remedy
Unshaven hair patches	Blunt razor	Change the blade or hone, and strop as necessary
	Incorrect skin tension	Stretch the skin smoothly before shaving
	Incorrect razor angle	Use the correct cutting angle
	Poor lathering	Re-lather in the required area; re-shave uneven areas
Shave not close enough	Strong beard growth	Complete a second-time-over shave and/or a sponge shave, as necessary
	Incorrect skin tension	Stretch the skin smoothly before shaving
	Incorrect razor angle	Use the correct cutting angle
	Poor lathering	Apply more lather and massage in upward moves
Shaving is painful	Blunt blade	Change the blade or hone, and strop as necessary
	Shaving dry	Apply lather, water or oil
	Shaving against the hair growth	Only shave *with* the hair growth on the first-time shave
Shaving rash (razor burn)	Shaving dry	Apply lather, water or oil
	Shaving against the hair growth	Shave *with* the hair growth
	Blunt razor	Change the blade or hone, and strop as necessary
	Shaving too close	Stop shaving
	Towels too hot	Remove and cool
Cuts to the skin	Blunt razor	Change the blade or hone, and strop as necessary
	Incorrect razor angle	Use the correct cutting angle
	Insufficient skin tension	Keep the skin taut
	Too much pressure applied on razor	Use light shaving strokes
Hair follicles inflamed	Ingrown hairs	Refer to a doctor if infected
Bumpy skin	Ingrown hairs	Advise the client to exfoliate their skin regularly to encourage the hairs to grow through and avoid shaving too close (particularly African-Caribbean men)
	Acne	Refer to doctor

Health and safety

Everyone in the salon has a duty to work safely and to keep the salon environment safe. This is particularly important when shaving because of the risk of cutting either the client's or your own skin, and the associated risk of cross-infection through open cuts. The following are some important factors that you must consider when providing shaving services.

Supervision

- Always work under expert supervision until you are competent.

Consultation

- If the client has any cuts or abrasions on his face, or if you suspect that an infection or infestation is present, you must not carry out the shave.

Safety and hygiene: general

- Use only clean towels, tools and equipment.
- When using a fixed-blade razor, make sure it is always sterilised before each use.
- When using a detachable-blade open razor, be sure to use a new blade for each new client.
- Always wear tight-fitting, surgical-type gloves whilst carrying out shaves. Try not to carry out any shaves if you already have cuts or abrasions on your hands.
- Special attention must always be given to hygiene when shaving, because of the risk of cross-infection through open cuts.

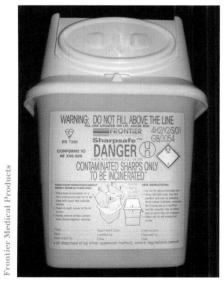

A sharps box

Safety and hygiene: sharps

- The use of fixed-blade razors is sometimes prohibited by local by-laws. Check the by-laws in your area before offering shaving services with this type of razor.
- Open and safety razors have very sharp blades. They must always be handled and used with great care.
- Always close the handle to protect the blade of an open razor when it is not being used or when it is being carried.
- *Never* place razors or other cutting tools in your pockets.
- Used razor blades, like all sharps, must be disposed of correctly in accordance with your salon's policy. Soiled disposable materials should be placed in sealed plastic bags for removal.

Accidents and injuries

- Make sure that you know the whereabouts of your salon's first-aid kit. Keep yourself up to date with your salon's first-aid and accident procedures.

- If the client's or your own skin is nicked during shaving, the bleeding may be stopped with styptic liquids or powders. (A *new* styptic pencil may be used instead, but it must then be discarded correctly: never reuse a styptic pencil.) Any soiled gowns or towels must be sealed in a plastic bag and laundered at a high temperature as soon as possible.

- If a more serious cut occurs, follow your salon's first-aid and accident procedures.

Methods of sterilisation

Sterilisation is the process of destroying *all* organisms, whether harmful or not. There are several methods of sterilisation available, which may be divided into the following groups.

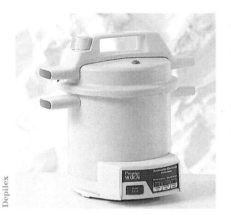

Depilex

An autoclave

Moist heat

Moist heat can be applied by boiling items in water for at least 20 minutes, or by immersing them in steam and under pressure in an autoclave.

Autoclaves are the preferred choice in many salons because they are the most effective method of sterilising tools. Items in autoclaves reach very high temperatures, so make sure that the tools are heat-resistant.

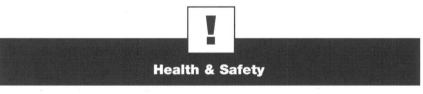

Health & Safety

Always take extra care when using an autoclave, and follow the manufacturer's instructions carefully.

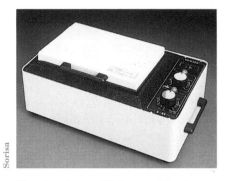

Sorisa

Dry heat sterilising cabinet

Dry heat

Dry heat is applied by placing items in an oven at very high temperatures. This method is most often used to sterilise sheets and towels, and is commonly used in hospitals. Some barbers use pre-packed towels which have been prepared in this way.

Ultraviolet rays

Tools can be sterilised in special cabinets using ultraviolet rays. These are popular in many salons as they are easy to use.

All tools must be *cleaned* thoroughly before they are placed in the cabinet, as ultraviolet rays will not work effectively if the tools are dirty. The tools must also be turned regularly so that all surfaces are exposed to the rays (for about 30 minutes on each surface). Ultraviolet ray cabinets are particularly good for *keeping* clean tools sterile.

An ultraviolet ray cabinet

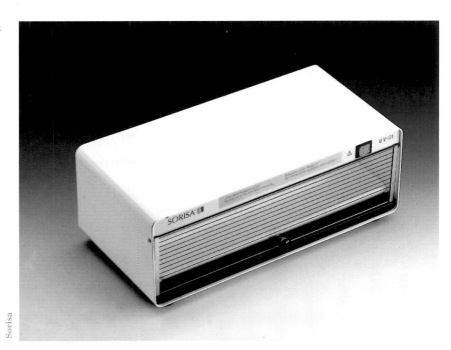

Sorisa

Vapours

Vapours are usually formaldehyde-based. They are used in cabinets, which are also popular in many salons because they too are easy to use. As with ultraviolet rays, all the tools must be cleaned thoroughly before they are placed in the vapour cabinet, as the vapours cannot work effectively if the tools are too dirty. The tools must be turned regularly to ensure that all surfaces are exposed to the vapours for about 30 minutes. Vapour cabinets are particularly good for keeping tools sterile once they have been cleaned.

Disinfectants

Disinfectants are effective only if they are used in the correct strength. In the barber's shop, tools are often stored in jars of disinfectant: note that the disinfectant is no longer effective when it has become soiled. Follow the manufacturers' instructions to ensure that disinfectants are used correctly.

Activities

1 Visit local barber's shops and use the Internet to research how professional shaving services are offered today and compare how they were offered in past times. Find out what type of clients request professional shaving services, the costs paid and whether face massage is also offered. Work out the reasons why the busiest salons are carrying out more shaving services. Consider whether your salon could do more to offer professional shaving and make recommendations to your manager. This activity may be combined with the activity in Chapter 12, 'Face massage'.

2 Contact the local council and use the Internet to research the local by-laws for your area. Find out whether any restrictions are placed on the use of fixed blade razors and what other requirements relate to barber's shops. Write up your findings and present them to your manager.

Check your knowledge

1 What are the factors that contributed to the decline of professional shaving services?

2 Explain the differences between wet and dry shaving methods.

3 Outline the importance of hair growth patterns when shaving.

4 What is the direction of shaving stroke for a first-time-over shave?

5 How should a client be prepared for shaving?

6 What is the correct way to pass an open style razor to another person?

7 What is the importance of local by-laws in relation to shaving services?

8 What type of razor is recommended for professional shaving services today?

9 What are the names of the two main types of fixed-blade razor?

10 List three key features required of a chair for use in professional shaving services.

11 Describe the correct use of a hone and strop.

12 What is the key requirement for preparing detachable-blade razors?

13 What are the purposes of hot and cool towels?

14 List four reasons for lathering prior to shaving.

15 What is the number and direction of shaving stroke for the top lip?

16 What is the direction of shaving stroke for a second-time-over shave?

17 Describe a sponge shave.

18 When would a cool towel not be applied after shaving services?

19 Why must gloves be worn when providing shaving services?

20 What actions should you take if you were to cut the client whilst shaving him?

21 What are the methods of sterilisation suitable for use in barber's shops?

12

Face massage

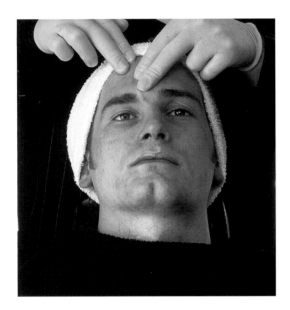

Learning objectives

Many men and women enjoy the relaxing effects of a face massage or facial. At one time the face massage was a popular service in many barber's shops, where it was often performed as part of the shaving service. The demand for face massage decreased, however, as more men started shaving at home and shaving in the barber's shop declined. More recently, though, and in common with shaving, there has been renewed interest in face massage as a service. Barbers are again offering face massage to their clients, who often request a massage at the time of their regular haircut.

This chapter looks at the traditional techniques used by barbers who provide face massage. It covers the following topics:

- **face massage – the effects and benefits**
- **consultation for face massage**
- **face massage products, tools and equipment**
- **face massage preparation**
- **preparing the face for massage – applying hot towels**
- **face massage techniques – including effleurage, petrissage, tapotement, friction and vibro massage**
- **a face massage routine**
- **finishing the face massage**
- **health and safety**

Face massage – effects and benefits

Face massage can be used to cleanse the skin and to improve its appearance, whilst providing a pleasant and enjoyable sensation for the client.

The effects and benefits of face massage include:

- cleansing and softening the skin, and removing dead epidermal skin cells
- increasing the supply of blood to the skin, to nourish the skin and to promote healthy muscles and a healthy skin colour
- stimulating and toning the underlying tissues, to help break down fatty deposits, to firm the muscles and to help define the natural contours of the face
- increasing the circulation of the lymphatic system, to help remove waste products and toxins from the skin
- stimulating or soothing of the nerves, depending on the massage technique being used
- relaxing the client, both physically and psychologically, thereby helping to relieve tension

The massage is usually performed with the hands, which manipulate the soft tissues of the face and neck. Sometimes a mechanical massager, commonly called a vibro massager, is also used. A range of different massage techniques can be used to produce either stimulating or relaxing effects, depending on the client's requirements and the area to be massaged.

Tip

Clients often enjoy having a face massage after shaving services. For weddings, some barbers offer shaving and face massage with haircutting and styling as a special service to the bridegroom and best man. Consider how you might offer these services to *your* clients.

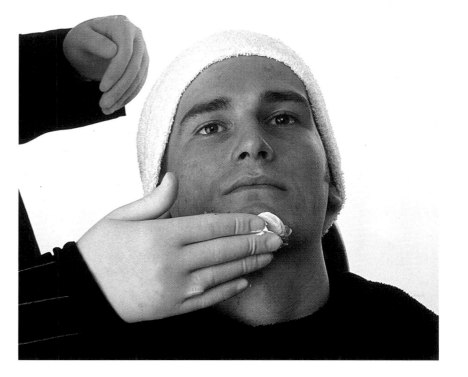

Anatomy of the face and neck

For safety, anyone with an interest in providing face massage *must* understand the basic anatomy of the face and the effects that massage has on its structures and systems. It is particularly important to know the position of the muscles and how they act, as the massage movements should generally be performed *along* the muscle and *towards its origin*. The position of the bones, nerves, blood supply and lymphatic system must all be understood, as they affect the choice of techniques and the speed and depth of pressure with which they are applied.

Bones

The bones are the foundation on which all the other structures and systems depend. The bones of particular interest in face massage are the maxillae, the mandible, the malar and the nasal bones. Other bones in the skull, known as the bones of the cranium, are also important in face massage, especially the frontal, the sphenoid and the temporal bones.

As you perform the face massage you will feel the bones beneath your fingers. In some areas of the face, such as on the forehead and around the eyes, the nose and the lips, there is little tissue between the bone and the surface of the skin. In these areas you must take care to choose the right massage technique and adjust both the speed and depth of pressure to avoid causing discomfort.

Bones of the face

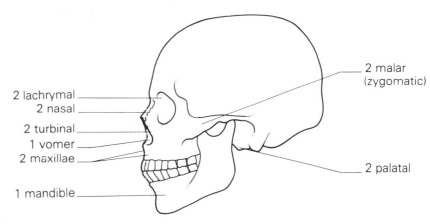

Bones of the cranium

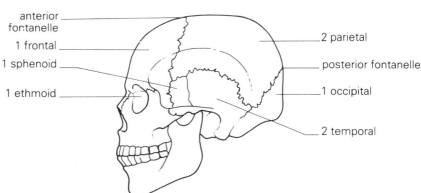

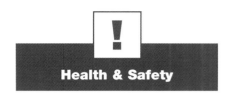

Health & Safety

If you wish to perform massage, it is important that you learn the position of muscles and their origins. Most massage movements are made along the muscle, *towards the origin* and *away from the point of insertion*. If you apply massage in the wrong places or in the wrong directions, you may cause the client discomfort.

Muscles

The muscles are an essential part of the face. They are interlinked with each other and with the bones to form an integrated system which allows you to eat, to speak, and to produce many different facial expressions.

Usually one end of the muscle is attached to a static bone by a strong tendon: this is called the muscle's origin. The other end is attached to a movable bone, to another muscle, or to the skin: this is called the muscle's insertion.

The main muscles of the face are:

- **occipital-frontalis** This muscle covers the top of the cranium. It enables you to lift the eyebrows, as when frowning.

- **orbicularis oculi** These muscles surround the eyes. They help to form the eyelids and allow the eyes to close.

- **orbicularis oris** This muscle surrounds the mouth and forms the lips. It allows you to close the mouth, and also helps in speaking.

- **temporalis** This muscle connects the temporal bone with the malar and mandible bones. It enables you to close the mouth and helps with chewing.

- **masseter** This muscle lies between the malar and mandible bones. It helps close the jaw during chewing.

- **zygomaticus** This muscle goes from the malar bones to the corners of the mouth. It allows the lip to move outwards (not shown in diagram).

- **sternomastoid** This muscle runs behind the ears to the temporal bones. It helps the head rotate and bow.

- **platysma** This muscle, within the front of the neck, allows you to wrinkle the skin and lower the corners of the mouth.

Muscles of the head and face

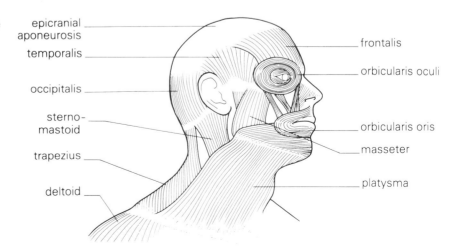

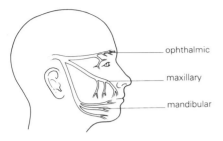

The 5th cranial (trigeminal) nerve

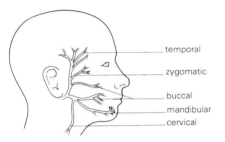

The 7th cranial (facial) nerve

Nerves

The nerves carry messages to and from the brain from and to all parts of the body.

In the face nerves carry messages to the skin, the muscles, the teeth, the nose and the mouth. The main nerves associated with the face are the 5th cranial nerve (the trigeminal nerve) and the 7th cranial nerve (the facial nerve).

Massage may be applied gently to the sites of nerve endings. During face massage, nerves may be either soothed or stimulated, depending on the technique used.

The blood supply

The heart pumps oxygenated blood through the arteries to nourish all areas of the body, including the face and head. The main blood supply to the face and head is through the carotid arteries, which divide into smaller arteries (arterioles) and then into many capillaries.

Eventually the capillaries join to form venules and then veins, which carry the blood back to the heart. The main veins from the face and head run down the sides of the neck, and are called the jugular veins.

Blood supply to the head

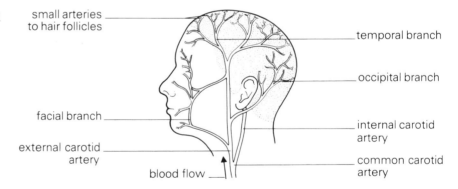

Blood vessels from the head

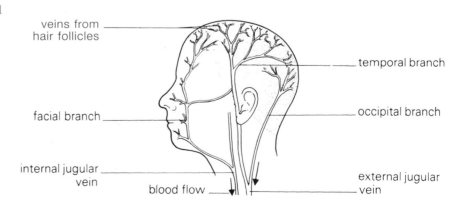

The heart pumps the oxygen-depleted blood to the lungs where the oxygen is replaced. The blood then returns to the heart, and the process starts all over again.

The blood supply can be stimulated by the application of face massage techniques (see page 239).

The lymphatic system

The structure of the lymphatic system is similar to that of the blood supply. It is made up of a network of lymph vessels, lymph nodes and lymph glands which closely follow the veins throughout the body.

Its main functions are to remove bacteria, foreign matter and excess fluids from the tissues. The lymphatic system is particularly important in helping to prevent infection, and is often triggered into response when an illness strikes. You may have heard the expression 'swollen glands' – or, indeed, experienced this painful condition yourself.

Lymph is a pale yellow fluid. Unlike the blood supply, the lymphatic system contains no pump. It is the movement of the larger muscles that forces lymph to move around the body. Lymph only travels away from the tissues towards the heart, not the other way.

Like the blood supply, the lymphatic system can be stimulated by the application of face massage techniques. Massage can help to promote the flow of lymph from the face and towards the lymph nodes, thereby removing waste products and toxins from the facial tissues.

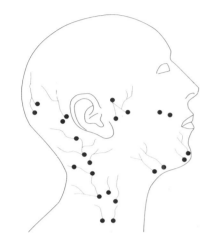

Lymph nodes

Consultation prior to face massage

A successful face massage will always begin with the consultation. Here you must identify your client's requirements and his reasons for wanting a face massage. It is particularly important that you assess whether the client is suitable for the massage to go ahead.

During the consultation you should discuss the client's expectations with him and provide advice on the actual results that he can expect. Take the time to explain what is involved, especially if this is the client's first face massage.

Here are some important factors that you must consider before providing a face massage:

- Make sure you establish what the client wants.
- Ask why the client wants a face massage – what are his expectations?
- Does the client have a moustache, a beard or large sideburns? Clients with long beards may not be suitable for face massage, as long beard hair is likely to pull during the massage and it is often difficult to perform the massage techniques effectively.

- Look for any signs of broken skin, abnormalities on the skin or any other contra-indications to carrying out the massage. Remember that the contra-indications may not always be obvious to the eye, so you should ask the client if he suffers from any skin disease or skin disorder, particularly allergies. Make sure you do this tactfully, and take care not to embarrass the client.

- Examine the skin to determine whether its condition is normal, dry or greasy. Discuss your findings with your client and agree on the most suitable products to use.

Contra-indications

Your examination of the skin will ensure that you identify any adverse conditions that may be present. It is particularly important to establish whether a suspected infection or infestation is present – if there is one, you must not carry out the face massage. (This area is covered more fully in Chapter 2, 'Client care for men'.)

Here are the most common contra-indications to face massage:

- broken or bleeding skin
- bruising, inflammation or swelling
- skin disorders, such as severe acne
- eye disorders, such as conjunctivitis
- skin diseases, such as impetigo

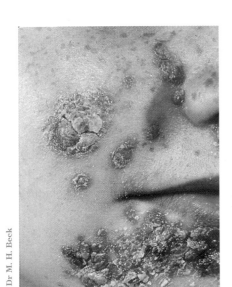

Impetigo

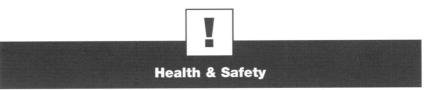

!

Health & Safety

If you see any contra-indications, especially any signs of broken skin, inflammation or disease, do not go ahead with the face massage. If you are unsure, seek help from a senior colleague and tactfully advise your client to see his doctor.

Acne

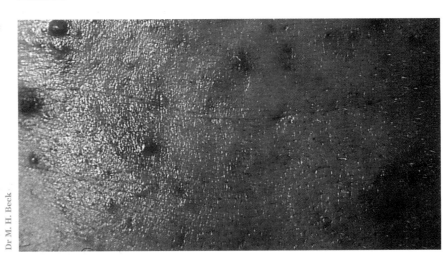

Products, tools and equipment

To provide face massage services you will need access to a range of products, tools and equipment.

Products

Cleansing creams are available for normal, dry and oily skin types. Massage creams are used as the massage 'medium', to lubricate the skin and to ensure that during the massage the hands can slide easily without dragging. There are many different kinds of massage cream available: choose the correct one for your client's skin type. Hypoallergenic products should be used where possible to avoid problems with clients who have allergies to ingredients such as perfumes.

Finishing products include astringents, which, because of their alcohol content, have a bracing and cooling effect on the skin. The cooling effect is caused by the evaporation of the alcohol from the skin. This makes the pores of the skin close and so reduces the risk of infection. Talcum powder may be used to ensure the skin is dry. It has a soothing and smoothing effect and can help to reduce the effect of shiny, oily skin.

Tools

You will need a sterile spatula or applicator for removing the massage cream from the tub and applying it to the face.

Equipment

You will need hot and cool towels, which should be sterilised if they are not specially supplied pre-packed. A face steamer may be used in place of the hot towels if preferred. If you wish to provide mechanical massage you will need a vibro machine and its applicators: some clients enjoy the intense sensation that this technique produces.

An adjustable chair should be available, which can be positioned so that the client can recline comfortably whilst the face massage is being carried out. If the chair does not have a headrest you must use some other suitable method of supporting the client's head. The height of the chair should be adjustable to avoid your having to bend uncomfortably (see page 207).

Tip

Exfoliating products are available that help remove the dead cells from the outer layer of skin. These can be useful for preventing ingrown hairs especially on African-Caribbean men.

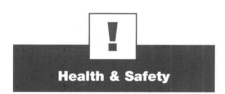

Health & Safety

Never place your fingers directly into the tub, as this would certainly contaminate the massage cream.

Tip

Remember to lock the chair before the client sits down to avoid accidents if the chair swivels.

Preparation for face massage

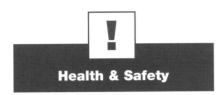

Health & Safety

Always ensure that the client's head is adequately supported throughout face massage services. Check that the client is comfortable, or harm may occur!

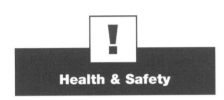

Health & Safety

Make sure your nails are not too long or they will catch the client's skin.

1   Carry out your consultation with the client. Look for signs of broken skin, abnormalities on the skin and any contra-indications. Determine the condition of the skin.

2   Agree with your client the massage techniques and products that you will use.

3   Before you begin work, gather together all the materials, products, tools and equipment you will require. Place them on a trolley so that you can work efficiently.

4   Position the client in a reclining chair with support for his head, using a clean paper towel over the headrest.

5   Gown the client and place a clean towel across his chest, tucking it in at the neck.

6   Place a second towel around the head to protect the hair and keep it from falling onto the face during the massage. To apply this, first fold it in half lengthways and then in half again. Then place the folded towel around the client's head, following the hairline across the forehead. Fold the ends of the towel under and place them between the client's head and the headrest to keep the towel in place.

7   Your hands and nails should be clean. Let your client see that you have washed your hands – make it clear that you have a high standard of hygiene in your work.

8   Remove any rings or bracelets that could scratch the client's skin before you commence the face massage.

Preparing the face for massage

Before the massage is carried out, you must ensure that the client's skin is cleaned of any visible signs of dirt and grease. It should be cleaned using a suitable cleansing cream.

1   Select a cleansing cream to meet the requirements of the client's skin.

2   Apply the cream using a circular motion. Start at the chin and work the cream up over the cheeks, then down the jawline and neck; follow up around the lips; go over the nose and around the eyes (taking extra care); and finally across the forehead.

3   Remove the cleansing cream with clean cottonwool or tissues. Use circular strokes in an upward and outward direction. If the client has a short beard or a moustache, ensure that it too is clean. (Remember that clients with long beards may not be suitable for face massage.)

A prepared client

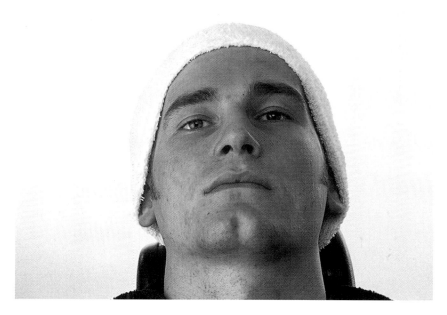

Applying hot towels

The facial muscles must now be relaxed and the skin pores opened. This is usually achieved by applying hot towels; a face steamer may be used if preferred.

Hot towels steam the face. In doing so, they help:

- to open the pores and remove dirt
- to lubricate the face, by stimulating the oil-producing glands
- to increase the flow of blood to the surface and relax the muscles, which makes massaging easier
- to relax the client

You must use *clean* towels. Some barbers use pre-packed towels, which are specially supplied ready-sterilised.

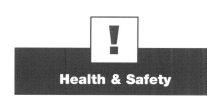

Health & Safety

Always test the temperature of the towel on the client's chin before wrapping to ensure that it is not too hot.

Be sure that the client's nose is not covered completely with the towel, as this would obstruct his airway.

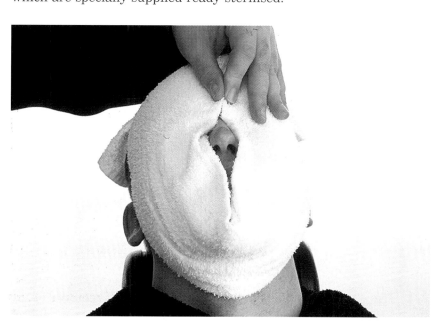

Hot towels are prepared in a steamer or by soaking them in hot water. Wring out the towel until it is nearly dry, then roll it up so that it retains its heat while you carry it to the client.

Unroll the towel and wrap it around the client's face, being careful not to cover the nose, so that the client can breathe. Allow the towel to cool.

The cool towel should be replaced by a second, and if necessary a third.

When using hot towels, remember the following important points:

- Always use clean towels for each new client.
- Prepare and apply the towels as quickly as possible but be sure to work safely – the quicker you are the more effective they will be.
- Avoid covering the client's nose.
- The towels should be nearly dry when they are applied.
- Remove the last hot towel before it becomes too cold – face massage should be performed on a warm, relaxed face!

Face massage techniques

Tip

Before you continue with a new massage movement, ask your client if the speed and pressure you are using are comfortable.

The face massage is performed using a variety of massage techniques, each of which produces a different effect. These techniques can be divided into two basic groups:

- manual massage
- mechanical massage

Manual massage techniques are performed with the hands and are used in virtually all face massages, and in most other massages too. Mechanical massage techniques require the use of a vibro machine: this imitates some of the manual massage movements, but its effect is often more intense. The vibro machine may be used on its own but is more often used in conjunction with manual massage techniques for clients who like the intense sensation that it creates.

All massage techniques should be adapted to suit the needs of the client and the area that is to be massaged. Both the speed of the technique and the depth of pressure applied may be adapted.

Remember that extra pressure should be applied only when working on the larger muscle areas.

Health & Safety

Take extra care when applying massaging techniques around the eyes, nose, temples, throat and lips. Do not use tapotement or vibro techniques on the nose, throat or lips – the intense movement would be very uncomfortable and might cause harm. **Never apply massage techniques directly to the eyes and ensure that you use light pressure and movements on other sensitive areas.**

Manual massage

Effleurage

Effleurage is a circular, stroking movement. It is the foundation of all good massage and is used to induce relaxation, particularly at the start and the completion of the face massage. It is also used as a link between the different massage techniques, to maintain the sensation of continual massage for the client.

The depth of pressure that you apply must be adapted to take account of the thickness of the underlying tissues.

The movement should be light, slow and rhythmical, so as to promote a sense of relaxation.

The main effects of effleurage are:

- relaxation of the muscles
- relaxation of the client
- increased circulation of the blood supply
- increased circulation of the lymphatic system

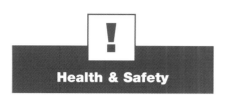

Health & Safety

The pressure should never be too deep, or discomfort and harm might occur.

Effleurage

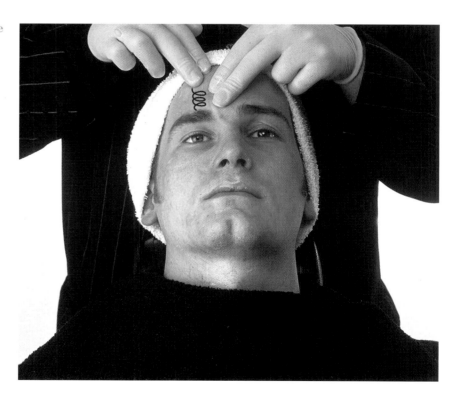

Petrissage

Petrissage is performed through a mixture of *pinching*, *kneading* and *rolling* movements. It is applied with both hands, which often work together to gently lift the skin between the fingers and thumbs, where it is squeezed, rolled and pinched with a gentle but firm pressure. These movements are repeated around the fuller parts of the face in a rhythmical and systematic pattern.

Petrissage

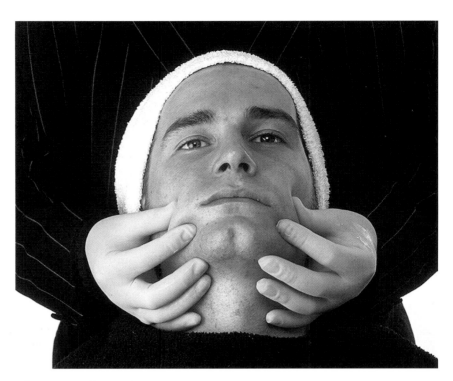

The main effects of petrissage are:

- toning of the muscles and the breakdown of fatty deposits in the tissues
- stimulation of the sebaceous glands
- increased circulation of the blood supply
- increased circulation of the lymphatic system

Tapotement

Tapotement

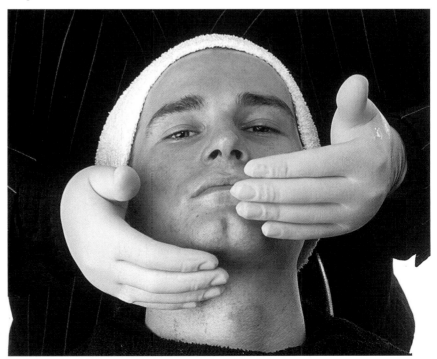

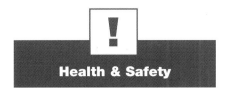

Health & Safety

Great care is needed when applying tapotement in areas with little underlying tissue, such as the forehead, eyes and lip areas.

Tapotement, or percussion, is the gentle *tapping* of the skin with the padded part of the fingertips. It is applied with both hands in a rhythmical manner to induce a pleasant and stimulating effect.

The main effects of tapotement are:

- stimulation of the nerves, producing an invigorating sensation
- increased blood supply to the surface of the skin
- toning of the muscles and the breakdown of fatty deposits in the tissues

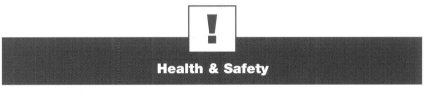

Health & Safety

Make sure that your fingernails are not too long before performing manual face massage, particularly when using tapotement, as long fingernails would dig into the skin.

Friction

Friction, or vibration, is applied to the site of the nerve endings or along the path of the nerves. It is performed by rapidly *vibrating* the fingers to produce a trembling movement, which is passed through the skin to the intended nerve.

Its main effect is:

- stimulation of the nerves, producing an invigorating sensation

Friction

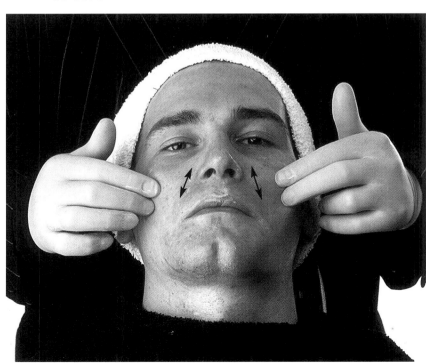

Mechanical massage

The vibro massage is a mechanical massage technique that imitates the manual massage movements of tapotement and friction.

The massage is performed with a vibrating machine, which has a range of different applicators for use on the scalp, face or body. A spiky applicator is provided for use on the scalp, whilst a sponge applicator and a rubber cup-shaped applicator are mostly intended for use on the face. Other applicators may also be provided for use on the larger areas of the body.

The effect produced by a vibro massager can be much more intense than that of manual techniques, and is not enjoyed by every client.

The vibro machine can be used in conjunction with the manual massage techniques or on its own: often it is not used at all. It is operated with both hands, one directing the movements whilst the other holds the machine firmly. It is most suitable for the fleshier parts of the face.

The main effects of vibro massage are:

- stimulation of the nerves, producing an invigorating sensation
- increased blood supply to the surface of the skin
- toning of the muscles and the breakdown of fatty deposits in the tissues

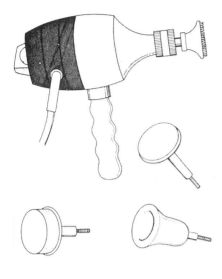

Vibro massager

Health & Safety

Vibro massage must *never* be used directly over delicate areas, such as around the eyes, nose, throat or lips.

Tip

To check that your client likes the effect of the vibro massage, first apply the technique to his arm before using it on the face.

A face massage routine

There are several different ways of performing a face massage. The starting place, the pattern of movements and the method of completion can all be tailored to suit the client and barber. Many barbers follow a preferred routine which they have developed through experience, and use their own creativity to make the massage more pleasurable and effective. With experience you too will begin to develop your own method of working.

A good face massage will always follow these simple rules:

- Each face massage must start and end with a relaxing massage movement, usually effleurage.
- The sequence of massage movements should flow logically so that the sensation created is one of continuous massage. For example, do not move your hands from one area to another, such as from the chin to the forehead, without linking the movement. Use broad, sweeping effleurage movements to link these areas together.

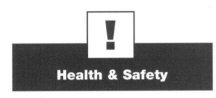

Tip

The face massage should be performed *before* the client's hair has been shampooed, cut or styled, otherwise the style will be ruined during the massage.

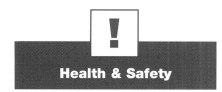

Health & Safety

If the face massage follows on from a shave and the skin has been nicked during shaving, you must ensure that any bleeding has stopped before providing the face massage. Gloves should then be worn but they must be tight-fitting, surgical-type gloves or you will not be able to perform the massage techniques effectively. Try to use latex-free gloves to avoid problems with clients who have allergies.

- Keep one or other of your hands in contact with the skin throughout the massage. Avoid any repeated stopping and starting, and try not to make jerky movements.
- Repeat each movement several times before moving on to the next area of the face.
- Ensure that you cover all areas of the face, unless your consultation has identified otherwise.
- Take your time. Your goal is to make the massage pleasant and relaxing: it is impossible to do this if you rush.

A manual face massage routine

The following routine is one example of how a face massage may be performed.

1 After the consultation ensure that your client is correctly gowned and protected.
2 Clean your client's face with cleansing cream.
3 Steam the face with two hot towels.
4 Apply sufficient massage cream to lubricate the face – do not apply too much or you will overload the skin. Starting at the chin, work the cream up over the cheeks, then down the jawline and neck (a). Follow up around the lips, go over the nose and around the eyes (taking extra care), and finally go across the forehead.
5 Standing behind the client, gently lift his chin to position the head for the massage.
6 Start the massage by sliding your fingers from the client's chin up the sides of the face to the temples. Without removing your hands from the face, place the pads of the first and second fingers of each hand on the sides of the forehead. Now gently move your fingers up and down between the hairline and the eyebrows whilst moving across the forehead towards the centre (b). Use light effleurage movements to relax the client, each hand moving in alternate directions (imagine you are drawing a zigzag pattern across the forehead). Work slowly and carefully to let the client become accustomed to the sensation.

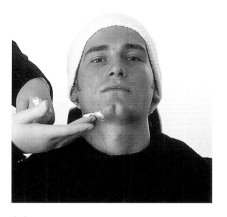

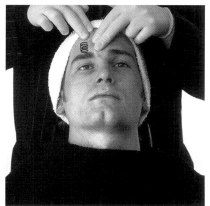

(a)   (b)

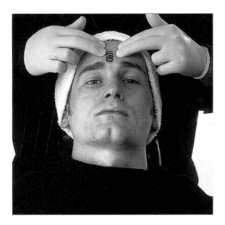

(c)

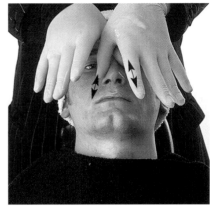

(d)

7 Move the fingers back towards the temples, then make small circular effleurage strokes up and down between the eyebrows and the hairline, working towards the centre of the forehead (c). *Repeat this series of movements at least once.*

8 Slide the fingers of both hands down the forehead to the bridge of the nose. Slide the thumbs across the bridge of the nose and cross them so that the thumb on the right hand is situated on the left side of the nose and the thumb on the left hand is situated on the right side of the nose. Using gentle pressure, slide the thumbs down and then back up the nose (d). Use slightly more pressure on the upward stroke. Take care not to depress the skin and actually block the nose. *Repeat this movement several times*, then uncross the thumbs at the top of the nose.

9 Slide your fingers down the sides of the nose and make spiralling effleurage movements across the cheeks, moving back up towards the temples (e). Slide your fingers gently under the eyes and back up to the top of the nose.

10 With each hand, place your middle finger on the eyebrow near the nose. Slide across the eyebrows towards the outer corners of the eyes. Slide down the sides of the cheeks to the corners of the mouth, and make spiralling movements back up the sides of the nose (f). *Repeat this series of movements at least once.*

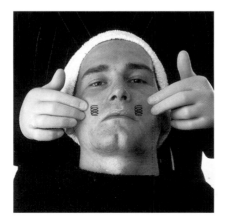

(e)

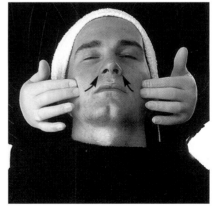

(f)

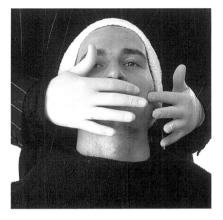

(g)

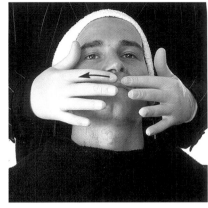

(h)

Tip

As noted, sometimes it is *necessary* to wear gloves, but you may choose to wear them at all times when you are carrying out face massage. This conforms to the highest standards of hygiene. Make sure you wear tight-fitting, surgical-type gloves or you will not be able to perform the massage techniques correctly. Try to use latex-free gloves to avoid problems with clients who have allergies.

A face massage should be a relaxing experience for the client: it must not be rushed. A typical face massage will take about 15–30 minutes to complete.

11 Slide your fingers back down the sides of the nose to the top lip. Place the index finger of your right hand flat against the top lip: the fingertip should be level with the left corner of the mouth (g). Gently slide the finger across the top lip keeping in contact with the skin (h). When the tip of the finger reaches the right corner of the mouth, replace it with the index finger of the left hand and make the same sliding movement in the other direction (i). *Repeat this movement several times, first one hand then the other, in a gentle rhythm.*

12 Slide the fingers down to the bottom lip, and repeat the same movements there.

13 Place the fingers on the chin. Using light pinching and squeezing petrissage movements, work up along the line of the jaw to the ear lobes (j, k). Slide the fingers back down the cheeks and to the corners of the mouth; then work back up towards the top of the ear, using the pinching movements as before. Make sure you cover all of the cheeks, but *do not go too close to the eyes*.

14 Slide back down to the corners of the mouth. Using the middle fingers of each hand make two deep, rotating petrissage movements, then continue this movement up across the cheeks and to the temples. Slide back to the chin. *Repeat the movement*, but this time finishing at the ear lobes.

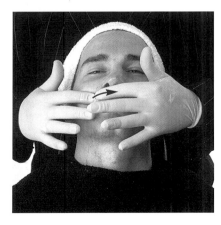

(i)

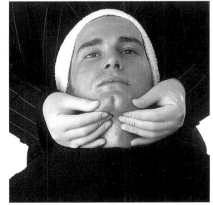

(j)

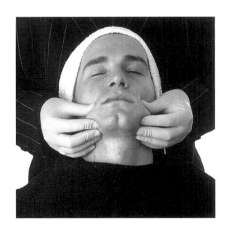

(k)

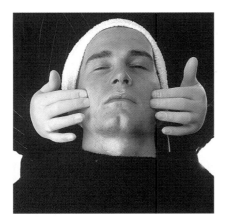

(l)

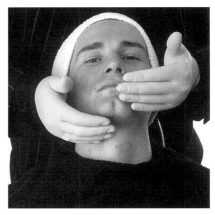

(m)

15 Slide your fingers back to the chin. Using your fingertips, apply a very light tapping tapotement movement and work up across the cheeks to the ear lobes and back to the corners of the mouth (l). *Repeat these movements* from the mouth up towards the temples (m). Develop a gentle rhythm to make the movement enjoyable.

16 Slide your fingers down the jawline back to the chin. Start on the lower lip and apply gentle rotating petrissage movements over the chin and down the neck, avoiding the Adam's apple. Cover the rest of the neck, working out from the chin (o).

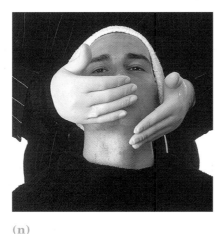

(n)

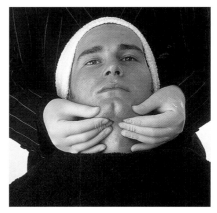

(o)

17 Complete the massage routine with gentle sweeping effleurage movements under the chin, across the neck and up over the cheeks.

18 Apply hot towels to remove all traces of the massage cream. Apply cool towels, an astringent, and talcum powder if required, and dry the face (see 'Finishing the face massage', page 248).

!

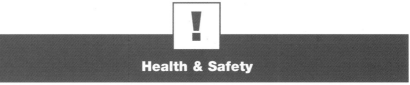

Health & Safety

Check that the client is comfortable at regular intervals, especially when commencing a new massage movement. Be alert to any non-verbal signs of discomfort shown by the client.

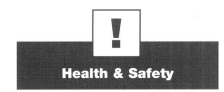

Health & Safety

Never use a vibro massager on the nose or around the eyes.

Tip

Little pressure is required when using a vibro massager on the face.

If the effects of a vibro massager are too strong, reduce them by placing your fingers on the client's face, and the cup on your fingers.

A vibro massage routine

The face massage may be completed with a vibro massager, used either on its own or in conjunction with the manual massage techniques. Before using it, make sure your client desires this form of massage. Confirm this by first testing the effect it produces on the client's arm.

The vibro should be used following the same pattern of movements used when applying the manual massage techniques it replaces. However, extra care must be taken, especially on bony areas like the forehead and jaw. Do not use it on the nose or around the eyes.

The rubber cup applicator is used for most face massage movements. It can produce intense, stimulating effects which some clients will not like. The sponge applicator has a more gentle and relaxing effect, and should be used after the massage cream has been removed.

Finishing the face massage

When the face massage is complete you should apply one or two final hot towels to remove all traces of the massage cream. Some clients enjoy the cooling and soothing effects of a cool towel: this is prepared and used just like a hot towel, but using cool water. Other clients even enjoy the bracing effects of a very cold towel, but you should ask before this is applied.

The effects of cool towels include:

- closing the pores of the skin, thereby reducing the risk of infection
- making the skin contract, producing a stimulating, invigorating sensation

A small amount of talcum powder may be applied to soothe and smooth the skin and to reduce any shiny effect that may have appeared. An astringent lotion may also be applied, if the client so desires. Astringent lotions have a bracing effect on the skin: as the alcohol in them evaporates, the skin cools, closing the pores of the face, and reducing the risk of infection.

When the face massage is complete, the client's hair should be shampooed, cut (if required) and styled.

Health and safety

Anyone providing face massage services has a duty to work safely and hygienically. You must maintain high standards of hygiene in all aspects of your work to minimise the risk of cross-infection.

The following are some important factors to consider when preparing to carry out a face massage.

Check for contra-indications

- Do not go ahead with the face massage if you see any contra-indications, especially any signs of broken skin, inflammation or disease. In these cases you should seek help from a senior colleague if necessary, and tactfully advise your client to see his doctor.

Use gloves as necessary

- If the face massage is following on from a shave and the skin has been nicked during shaving, make sure that any bleeding has stopped before providing the face massage. Wear tight-fitting, surgical-type gloves or you will not be able to perform the massage techniques effectively. Make sure you apply sufficient massage cream to lubricate the skin, as gloves can drag and pull the skin more easily. Try to use latex-free gloves to avoid problems with clients who have allergies.

Do not harm the client!

- Take extra care when applying massaging techniques around the eyes, the nose, the temples, the throat and the lip areas. *Do not use tapotement or vibro techniques in these areas*, as the intense movement will be very uncomfortable and may cause harm.
- *Never apply massage techniques directly to the eyes.* Use only light pressure and movements on any sensitive area. Be alert to any non-verbal signs of discomfort shown by the client.
- Keep your fingernails short. If they are too long they may catch the client's skin.

Maintain a high standard of hygiene

- Use only clean towels, tools and equipment.
- Always pay special attention to hygiene when providing face massage: your hands will be working close to the client's mouth, eyes and nose. Always wash your hands thoroughly before you begin work, and make sure you are maintaining high standards of personal hygiene.
- You may wish to observe the highest standard of hygiene by always wearing gloves when providing face massage services. If so, they must always be tight-fitting, surgical-type gloves.

Be prepared for accidents

- Make sure that you know the whereabouts of your salon's first-aid kit.
- Keep yourself up to date with your salon's first-aid and accident procedures.
- Re-read the section on methods of sterilisation in Chapter 2, 'Client care for men'.

Activities

1 Visit local barber's shops and use the Internet to research how face massage services offered today compare to those offered in past times. Find out what type of clients request face massage services, the costs paid and whether shaving is also offered. Work out the reasons why the busiest salons are carrying out more face massage services. Consider whether your salon could do more to offer face massage and make recommendations to your manager. This activity may be combined with the activity in Chapter 11, 'Shaving'.

2 Practice your face massage techniques on a colleague or mannequin head until the movements link together in a fluid, unbroken routine.

Check your knowledge

1 List six effects of face massage.

2 List the main bones of the face affected by face massage.

3 What is the muscle's insertion?

4 Describe the position and function of the orbicularis oris.

5 What are the main function of nerves?

6 Describe the blood supply to the face.

7 State two functions of the lymphatic system.

8 List five contra-indications to face massage.

9 What is the purpose of an astringent?

10 What piece of equipment is used to provide mechanical massage?

11 List four reasons for using hot towels prior to a face massage.

12 Why is a head rest important when providing face massage services?

13 List the main effects of the petrissage massage movement.

14 Which manual massage movement is used to stimulate the nerve endings?

15 State where mechanical massage techniques must not be applied.

16 Why must gloves be worn when providing face massage immediately after shaving services?

17 Describe how the barber's hands and nails should be prepared before providing face massage services.

18 Explain the course of action required if you suspect contra-indications are present.

19 Why should latex-free gloves be used for face massage wherever possible?

Designing facial hair shapes

13

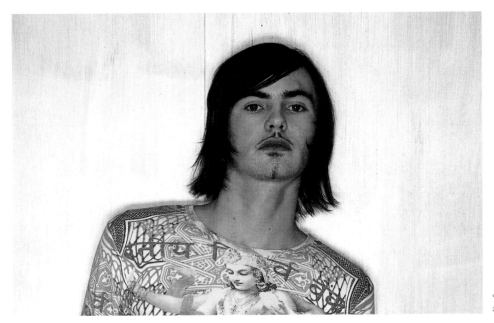

Forfex

Learning objectives

Whilst longer beards and moustaches are now seldom worn, the popularity of shorter beard and moustache shapes has continued to grow. Modern men are now often choosing to wear shorter facial hair shapes to suit their highly personalised short haircuts. But fashions often change and longer hairstyles could see longer beard shapes returning. The barber must be prepared for such events as the beard or moustache is again playing an important role in establishing an individual look for many men.

In this chapter we will be looking at the techniques used for designing and creating facial hair shapes and will be covering the following topics:

- **factors to be considered when designing a variety of facial hair shapes**
- **traditional, contemporary and emerging beard and moustache shapes**
- **cutting procedures**
- **notes on health and safety**

Before reading this chapter it may help you to read Chapter 4, 'Cutting facial hair using basic techniques'.

Factors to be considered when designing a variety of facial hair shapes

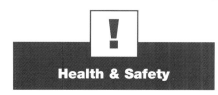

Health & Safety

You must carry out a thorough consultation to ensure that you identify any adverse conditions of the hair or skin that may be present. It is particularly important to establish whether a suspected infection or infestation is present, as this would prevent you from cutting the facial hair. (This area is covered more fully in Chapter 2, 'Client care for men').

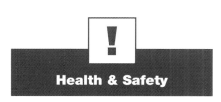

Health & Safety

Take extra care when cutting very coarse or dense beards, as the hair is liable to fly in all directions while it is being cut. Make sure the client's eyes are well protected with clean cotton wool pads or tissues and keep your face well away from the work. If you find the hair is very strong and springy you may have to wear safety glasses to protect your eyes!

There are many similarities between maintaining an existing beard or moustache shape and designing and creating new shapes. The same cutting techniques can be used for most of the work required and, of course, the shapes produced often have styling features that are similar. Factors including the hairstyle, head and face shape, hair density and adverse hair and skin conditions still have to be fully considered. But differences do exist in the level of consultation required (establishing the factors is even more important when designing new facial hair shapes), and in the methods that are used to achieve the new shapes.

The principles learnt earlier about shape and form are also more important when designing a new facial hair shape, as you are starting with what might be called a blank canvas. But, as with advanced haircutting, here too the principles are applied more loosely where required by the hairstyle, facial hair shape and overall look. The work undertaken regularly requires cutting techniques to be combined and adapted to take account of both the client's wishes and the many factors that affect the creation of the new shape. The client consultation is essential in designing and personalising the right shape for each client.

Consultation – designing the correct shape

Before you design a new beard or moustache shape you must carry out a thorough consultation to consider factors including the client's wishes, face shape and hairstyle. Here is a reminder of some of the critical factors that must be considered when designing and creating facial hair shapes:

- accurately establish what the client wants
- determine why he wishes to have a beard and/or moustache shape
- look for signs of broken skin, abnormalities on the skin, or any unusual facial features or beard growth patterns
- is the beard hair fine, medium or coarse?
- is the beard growth dense or sparse – does the density of beard growth vary around the face?
- determine the client's face shape
- determine the length and shape of his hairstyle

Tip

Remember to look for variations in the density of growth when designing beard shapes. The hair may have to be left long in some areas to cover very sparse growth or a scar, while at other times sparse growth may mean that some shapes cannot be grown at all!

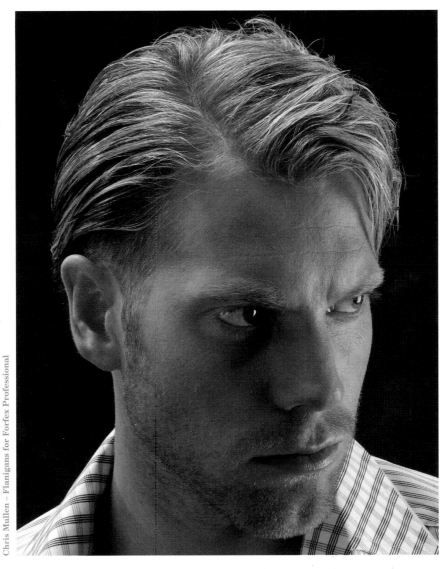

Chris Mullen – Flanigans for Forfex Professional

Tip

Hair growth patterns must be identified because they determine both the shape that can be created and the techniques that you should use. Some clients have very strong hair growth patterns in their beard, such as hair whorls, which should be cut by following the direction of hair growth around the whorl.

Face shape, facial features and hairstyle

The client's face shape and facial features must be considered when choosing the most suitable shape for each client. The size and position of the mouth, width of the top lip, shape of the nose, jaw and chin and presence of any unusual features, such as moles, dimples, scarring or facial piercings must all be established.

Different face shapes require different beard and moustache shapes. Here are some examples:

Tip

Remember, a *full beard* covers the whole area of beard and moustache growth on the face, though this may be outlined. A *partial beard* is any beard where part of the beard or moustache growth inside the natural outline is removed.

Facial shape	*Beard and moustache shape*
A round face	Choose a beard shape that is longer at the chin to make the face appear longer and less round. Keep the sides short and avoid bushy sideburns, as they will make the face appear more round. Partial beards, such as a goatee or full beards like a King Edward beard are often good shapes to choose.
A large face	A larger moustache shape is usually more suitable, as a small moustache will appear lost and will make the face appear bigger. The width of the top lip must also be considered because a large moustache would appear too big on a narrow lip. Small, partial beards can also appear lost, so consider large partial or full beards.
A small face	The smaller face is more suited to smaller beard and moustache shapes, such as a modern goatee.
A long face	Choose a beard shape that is fuller at the sides and shorter at the chin. This will help to make the face appear less long. Make sure any change in length is gradual so as not to be obvious.
A square face	Full beard shapes are often more suitable, which should be shorter at the sides and longer towards the chin.
An oval face shape	Almost any beard shape is suitable, but you must take into account the client's hairstyle.

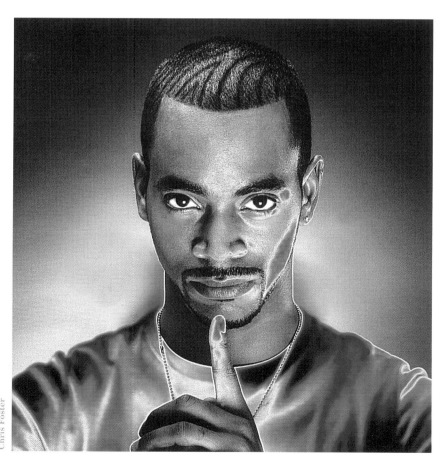

Chris Foster

Tip

If your client has male pattern baldness avoid longer and fuller shapes, especially if their hairstyle is cut short. Closer cut beards and moustaches usually work best as they are evenly balanced with such haircuts.

Tip

Make sure that the neck outline is cut slightly higher in the centre than at the sides to compensate for the head being positioned back at an angle during cutting, or the outline will appear longer in the centre when the head returns to the normal position.

The length and shape of the client's hairstyle are important factors affecting the design of the facial hair shape. Longer hairstyles tend to suit longer, fuller beard shapes as shorter shapes can appear unbalanced, but care must be taken not to 'overpower' the client's face, head and body shape with too much hair! Likewise, shorter beard shapes often work best with shorter hairstyles.

Cutting facial hair outlines

Most men have dense hair growth that grows outside the natural beard hairline. Shorter layered beard shapes should always be outlined and the unwanted hair from outside the outline removed or the beard will appear unfinished. In longer beards it can seem less important, as the longer hair may cover the outline, but unwanted hair outside the outline should still be removed for the result to

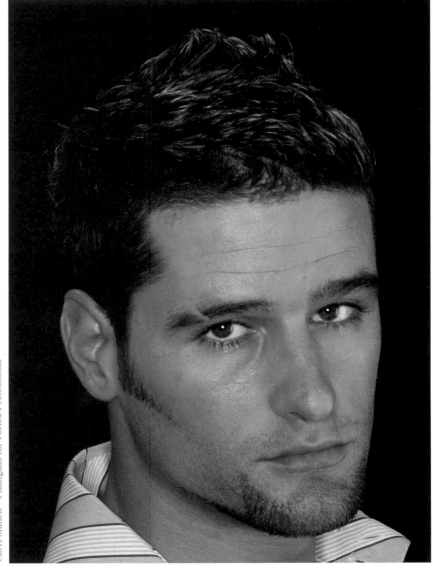

Chris Mullen – Flanigans for Forfex Professional

Tip

To ensure that the outlines of the beard and moustache are cut level place the thumb of one hand on the outline of one side of the face at the required position. Whilst looking in the mirror slide the other thumb down to the same position on the outline of the other side of the face until both thumbs appear level. Memorise the position of the thumbs; you can use a position on the face between the ear, eye and nose as a point of reference. Now cut each outline to the correct position and length. This method can be easily adapted to establish the width of the beard or moustache and so obtain symmetrical shapes, even in the most elaborate designs.

appear professional. The outlines may be cut to give a natural appearance, or they may be created with lines that are more obvious.

Strong, less natural outlines may be features of some shapes and in such cases the outlines can be cut to almost anywhere, or even incorporated into elaborate patterns and designs (see Chapter 14, 'Design and create patterns in hair').

Tramlines and channelling can be added to the beard and moustache design. These can range from simple 2D shapes to complex geometric designs and sometimes 3D effects are included. But most often it is simple tramlines that are used in facial hair designs.

Usually men want facial hair shapes that are less radical, with the emphasis on creating a natural balanced look that matches their haircut. In each case the face shape and hairstyle should be used to determine the correct choice of shape for each client. Here are some important things to remember about designing facial hair shapes:

- Many facial hair shapes are improved by having distinct outlines. Outlines help to define and balance the beard or moustache shape.
- Avoid cutting into the beard or moustache outline unless the look requires these more radical and less natural effects.
- Beard and moustache outlines should usually be cut level, unless the look is to be asymmetric. Do not use the ears or eyes to determine the level of the outlines, as they are not usually level themselves. (See Tip).
- Pay particular attention to where the beard meets the haircut and ensure that they blend together, as required.
- Consider the sideburns when cutting moustache and partial beard shapes and ensure that they compliment each other.
- Think of the haircut and moustache and/or beard as being integrated parts of one style.

Traditional and contemporary beard and moustache shapes

Chapter 4 describes how many traditional beard and moustache shapes have developed over the years. Many of these shapes were named after the men who wore them at different times, such as the King Edward, which means that similar shapes were sometimes known by different names, e.g. the Van Dyke is similar to the King Edward. Some shapes were adopted by men in certain roles and acquired names to reflect this, such as the military moustache. Other shapes were popular with men in different social classes, e.g. in the early 1900s few working class men would wear a

King Edward beard. Yet other shapes were popular in certain countries and were referred to by the country involved, e.g. the French Fork.

Some traditional shapes are still current or popular today and are usually referred to by their traditional name. Other newer, contemporary shapes do not often acquire specific names and are simply described by the shape formed, or by reference to a similar traditional shape. This can make identification of newer shapes difficult, so care must be taken to make sure the right shape has been chosen before commencing work. Reference to photographs or sketches is essential during the consultation for creating a new facial hair design.

Here is a selection of traditional and contemporary beard and moustache shapes to provide some ideas for your own designs and examples of some names used to describe them. Remember, any of the traditional shapes could become fashionable and would then also be referred to as being current.

Traditional beard shapes

- King Edward
- Norris Skipper
- Balbo
- Goatee
- The Spade
- Old Dutch
- Chin Curtain
- Imperial
- Friendly Mutton Chops
- French Fork

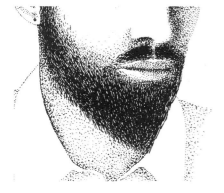

King Edward

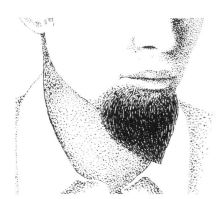

Norris Skipper

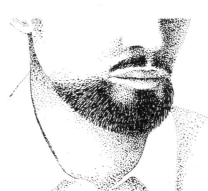

Balbo

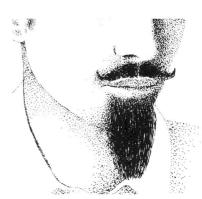

Goatee

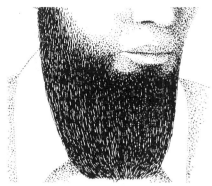

The Spade

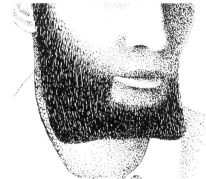

Old Dutch

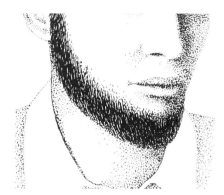

Chin Curtain

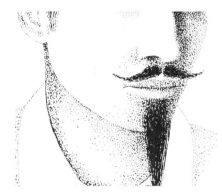

Imperial

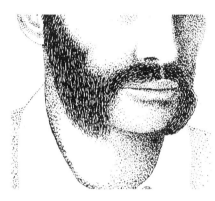

Friendly Mutton Chops

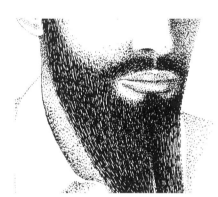

French Fork

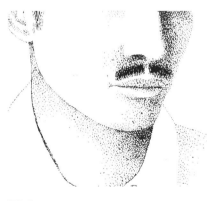

Major

Traditional moustache shapes

- Major
- Regent
- Military
- Chaplin or Square Button
- Old Bill
- Walrus
- Mexican
- Pencil Line
- Howie
- Box Car

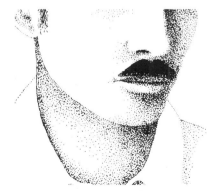

Regent

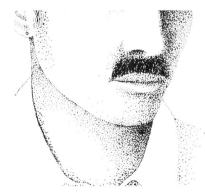

Military

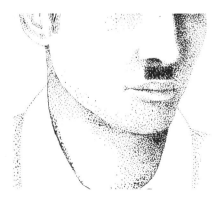

Chaplin or Square Button

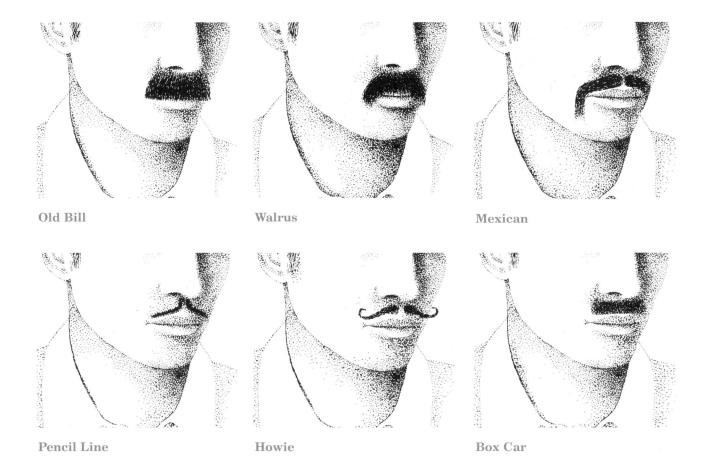

Old Bill

Walrus

Mexican

Pencil Line

Howie

Box Car

Contemporary beard and moustache shapes

- Modern Goatee Beard
- Cropped Modern Norris Skipper Beard
- Short Chin Cap Beard

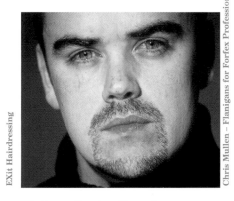

Modern Goatee Beard

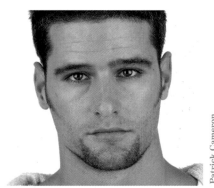

Cropped Modern Norris Skipper Beard

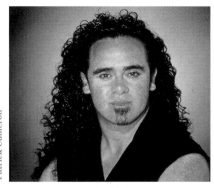

Short Chin Cap Beard

EXit Hairdressing

Chris Mullen – Flanigans for Forfex Professional

Patrick Cameron

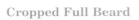

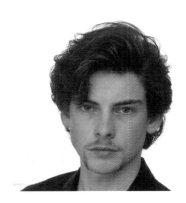

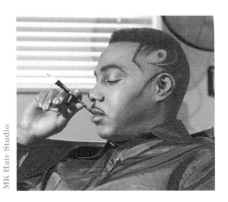

Cropped Full Beard

Thin Mexican Moustache

Modified Pencil Line
Moustache

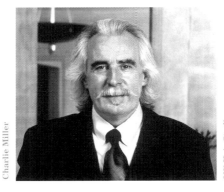

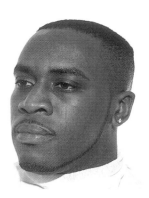

Colonel Moustache

Pencil Line Chin Curtain and
Moustache

- Cropped Full Beard
- Thin Mexican Moustache
- Modified Pencil Line Moustache
- Colonel Moustache
- Pencil Line Chin Curtain and Moustache

Emerging beards and moustaches

Emerging beard and moustache shapes are developed as barbers
consider the latest hairstyles and design beard and moustache
shapes that compliment the looks required. This often involves
combining and adapting traditional and new beard shapes with
traditional and new moustache shapes. These shapes are then
amended and other newer ideas are added, such as tramlines, in
order to create the unique looks required. Many emerging shapes
are first seen in magazines and at trade shows and exhibitions.
Competitions are also good places to see and develop ideas for
emerging beard and moustache shapes.

Cutting procedures

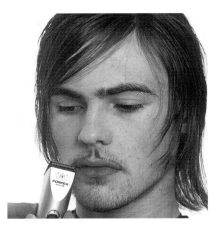

(a) Step 4

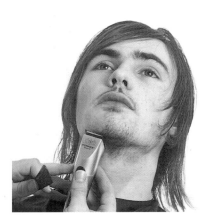

(b) Step 7

Current moustache and beard shapes

Jordan – pencil line modified imperial moustache and beard

1 Start at one side of your client and begin cutting the beard hair to the correct length using the scissors- or clippers-over-comb technique.

2 Repeat this on the other side.

3 Move to the centre of the beard and blend the two sides together to create an even, continuous effect.

4 Move to one side of the moustache. Carefully outline the moustache along the top lip to create the required shape with the tips of your scissors or with the clippers.

5 Repeat this on the other side of the moustache.

6 Using your comb, lift small sections of the moustache hair and cut this to the required length.

7 Carefully establish the outline for the pencil line beard shape and cut the outline to the correct position.

8 Cut the other outlines on the cheeks, chin or above the moustache, as required. Refer to the mirror to keep the outlines symmetrical.

9 Remove unwanted hair from outside the outlines, as required.

10 Shave the areas outside the outlines if required (see Chapter 11).

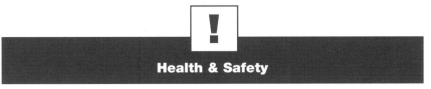

Health & Safety

Remove excess hair cuttings from the client's face and neck at regular intervals to ensure he is comfortable.

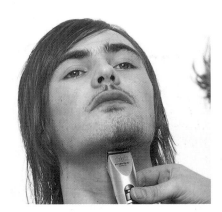

(c) Step 7

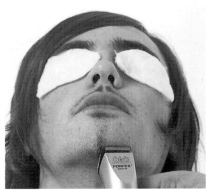

(d) Step 8 – eye protection applied whilst removing main growth

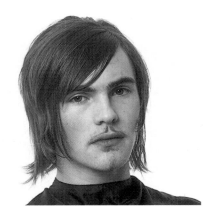

(e) The finished look

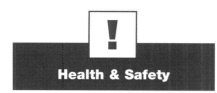

Adam – short traditional Mexican

The client is a model who has grown a basic moustache shape for his role in a forthcoming TV advertisement.

1 Move to one side of the moustache. Carefully outline the moustache along the top lip to create the required shape with the tips of your scissors or with the clippers.

2 Repeat this on the other side of the moustache.

3 Using your comb, lift small sections of the moustache hair and cut this to the required length.

4 Carefully establish the outline for the moustache shape and cut the outline to the correct position.

5 Cut the other outlines on the cheeks, chin and above the moustache, as required. Refer to the mirror to keep the outlines symmetrical.

6 Remove unwanted hair from outside the outlines, as required.

7 Shave the areas outside the outlines if required (see Chapter 11).

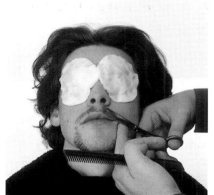

(a) Step 1

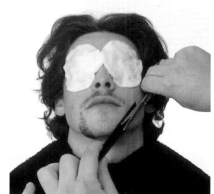

(b) Step 3

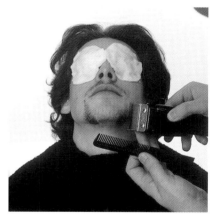

(c) Step 4

Tip

Outlines can be achieved by cutting the hair with either close-cutting clippers or an electric razor. The outline hair may also be removed completely by shaving with a razor, which should be used following the shaving procedure described in Chapter 11.

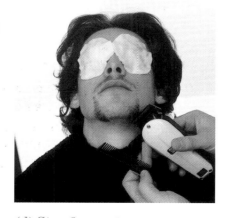

(d) Step 6

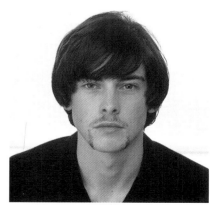

(e) The finished look

Health and safety

Everyone in the salon has a duty to work safely and keep his or her environment safe. It is important to consider health and safety when cutting facial hair because of the risks associated with using electricity, the risk of cutting the skin and the risk of hair cuttings entering the eyes. Here are some important health and safety factors that you must consider when providing hair cutting services:

- If the client has any cuts or abrasions on their face, or you suspect that an infection or infestation is present, the work must not be carried out.

- Pay special attention to hygiene when cutting facial hair because of the risk of cross-infection through open cuts.

- Always protect the client's eyes from hairs with tissues or cotton wool pads. Keep your own face away from your work; wear safety glasses for protection.

- Open and safety razors have very sharp blades and must always be handled and used with great care.

- Always close the handle to protect the blade of an open razor when it is not being used or when it is being carried.

- *Never* place razors or other cutting tools in pockets.

- A fixed-blade razor must always be *sterilised* before each use.

- A new blade must always be used for each new client when using a detachable blade open razor.

- Used razor blades, called sharps, must be disposed of correctly in accordance with your salon policy. Soiled disposable materials should be placed in sealed plastic bags for removal.

- Electrical equipment must always be handled and used with care in accordance with the manufacturer's instructions.

- *Never* use or place electric clippers or other electrical equipment near water.

- *Do not* go near electrical equipment that is lying in water – isolate the mains power first.

- Visually check that electrical equipment is safe to use before commencing work – check that the cable has not frayed or been pulled and that the plug is not loose.

- Pay attention to the position of cables when using and storing electrical equipment.

- *Never* overload sockets by plugging too many items of electrical equipment into the same socket.

- Follow the manufacturer's instructions for the care of your clippers – ensure that you clean and lubricate the blades regularly to avoid damage.

- Only use clean tools and equipment.

- Make sure that you know the whereabouts of your salon's first-aid kit. Keep yourself up to date with your salon's first-aid and accident procedures.

- Electrical equipment must be regularly tested and given a certificate of testing to confirm that it is safe for use. Your salon owner will ensure that this is carried out, as required.

Activity

Use the Internet and magazines to find images that show how men are currently wearing beards and moustaches and what new shapes are emerging. Use this information to design and create some new shapes. Photograph the created shapes – remember to get permission from your manager and clients before taking their photographs. Use all the images to produce a style book that can be used during consultation with clients in your salon. Remember to get permission from your manager before using the style book.

Check your knowledge

1 When might you need to design a beard shape that is left longer in certain areas?

2 List techniques that can be used to incorporate patterns into beard and moustache designs.

3 How should the neck outline be cut to ensure that it appears level?

4 Why is it important to consider the hairstyle when designing a new beard and moustache shape?

5 Describe the beard and moustache shape most suited to a client with a small face.

6 Why is it important to consider existing sideburns when designing a new moustache shape?

7 What differences would facial piercing make to the design and creation of a new beard shape?

8 Sketch a traditional military moustache shape.

9 Describe two traditional beard shapes.

10 List two current beard and moustache shapes.

11 Describe how emerging beard and moustache shapes are developed.

12 What action should be taken if the client has an open cut on his face?

13 How should hair clippings be disposed of?

14 Why is it important to not plug too many items of electrical equipment into one socket?

Design and create patterns in hair

14

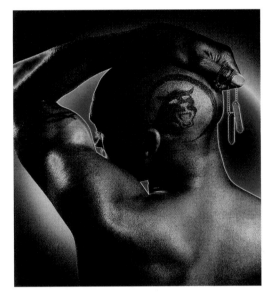

Chris Foster

Learning objectives

In the 1970s some men, and boys, wore short haircuts that were personalised by the addition of simple lines and patterns. One of the most popular of these haircuts was the 'tennis ball crew-cut', where all of the hair was cut to about 10 mm in length and a curved tramline was added to make the head resemble a tennis ball. Other short haircuts, especially on African-Caribbean hair, had partings channelled into the hair to make them appear more interesting. Sometimes simple patterns, shapes or words were created, often representing a favourite sports team or club. But recently much more elaborate patterns are being created in both haircuts and facial hair. Two-dimensional (2D) and three-dimensional (3D) designs can be added and complex compositions produced that are perhaps better described as 'works of art'.

In this chapter we will be looking at the techniques used for designing and creating patterns in hair and will be covering the following topics:

- **factors to be considered when designing and creating patterns in hair**
- **principles of design – including shape and form, scale, freehand work and the use of stencils, proportion and position**
- **cutting techniques – including channelling, tramlines and razoring**
- **cutting procedures**
- **notes on health and safety**

Before reading this chapter it may help you to read Chapter 5, 'Cutting men's hair using basic techniques' and Chapter 10, 'Advanced men's hair cutting'.

Factors to be considered when designing and creating patterns in hair

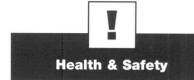

Health & Safety

You must carry out a thorough consultation to ensure that you identify any adverse conditions of the hair or skin that may be present. It is particularly important to establish whether a suspected infection or infestation is present, as this would prevent you from cutting the hair. (This area is covered more fully in Chapter 2, 'Client care for men').

Tip

Hair growth patterns must be identified because they determine the shapes that can be created and the techniques that you should use. The movement created by the hair growth pattern can become a feature of the design and be incorporated into the pattern to create a particular effect.

Tip

Remember to look for variations in the density of growth when designing the pattern. The design may have to be adapted in some areas to cover very sparse growth or a scar.

Many similarities exist in the procedures used to create regular haircuts and create haircuts with patterns. The same cutting techniques can be used for most of the work required and some of the basic haircut shapes produced are the same. The head and face shape, hair density, adverse hair and skin conditions and other factors still have to be fully considered. But differences do exist in the consultation required (accurately establishing what design the client wants is especially important when the patterns can be very obvious), and in some of the techniques used.

The work regularly requires cutting techniques to be combined and adapted to take account of both the client's wishes and the many factors that affect the creation of the new pattern. The client consultation is essential in designing and personalising the right shape for each client.

Consultation

Before you can design or create the pattern you must carry out a thorough consultation to consider factors including the client's wishes, face shape and existing haircut. Here is a reminder of some of the critical factors that must be considered when designing and creating patterns in hair:

- accurately establish what the client wants
- determine why he wishes to have a pattern in his hair
- look for signs of broken skin, abnormalities on the skin, or any unusual features or hair growth patterns
- is the hair fine, medium or coarse?
- is the hair growth dense or sparse – does the density of hair growth vary around the head and face?
- determine the client's face shape
- determine the existing and required length and shape of his hairstyle

Face shape, features and haircut length

The client's face shape and features must be considered when choosing the most suitable haircut and pattern. The principles applied to choosing the right shape and length of haircut for different face shapes is explained fully in Chapter 5, 'Cutting men's hair using basic techniques' and they also apply here. But an additional concern when creating patterns in hair is the existing and required length of the haircut.

The length of the client's existing haircut is an important factor because some patterns cannot be achieved if the hair is too short, e.g. 3D effects cannot be created easily on hair layers shorter than 5 mm. Longer haircuts with layers beyond around 4 cm in length can of course be shortened to lengths suitable for creating patterns, but

Tip

On clients with male pattern baldness closer cut haircuts usually work best as the foundation for the pattern because they appear more evenly balanced.

clients who wish to keep their hair layers longer than this should be discouraged from including patterns in these areas. Patterns may be included in other shorter areas though, such as in the back and sides even though the layers on the top are longer. Longer layers are less suitable for creating patterns because the hair tends to cover the pattern and the effect can appear unbalanced. Shorter, layered haircuts between 5 mm and 2 cm are usually best for 2D designs and geometrical shapes, but layers up to 4 cm often work better for 3D designs, as the thickness makes creating the 3D effect easier. Pictorial patterns too work well on hair this length. On hair shorter than 5 mm good pictorial, graphical or geometric shapes can be created.

Principles of design

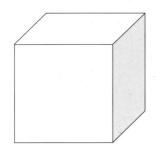

2D shape

The basic principles used when designing patterns in hair are:

- shape and form
- scale
- proportion
- position

Shape and form

Shape describes a two-dimensional or 2D object. Form refers to the appearance of the 3D effect, or depth of an object. Shape and form both define the exterior outline shape of the overall pattern to be created and the outline shapes of each individual object within the pattern. The most important element of any shape or form is the line. Lines come in many different varieties – fine lines, thick lines, broken lines, etc. They are used to determine the placing of the object and to create precise limits on the space between objects within the pattern. When creating complex designs any complicated shapes are usually broken down into simple geometric shapes that can be more easily created. They are then joined together when the composition is complete.

3D shape

When creating patterns in hair, the lines are created using either a freehand technique with electric clippers, trimmers or scissors, or by following the outline of a stencil, which may have been designed by the barber or purchased ready made.

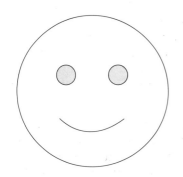

A simple stencil

Scale

Usually the objects that inspire designs are bigger or smaller than the size of pattern we wish to create. This means the design of the object must be enlarged or reduced and we use scale to help us do this. Scale is a number system that allows us to establish the relative dimensions of objects and designs. In this way an object that is 20 cm × 10 cm can be reduced to half its original size by dividing each measurement by two, making the new size 10 cm × 5 cm. This design would be a 1:2 scale replica of the original object.

Tip

To ensure that the lines of the pattern are cut accurately when using freehand techniques place the thumb of one hand on the line of one object within the design. Stand back at arm's length, or looking in the mirror, slide the other thumb to the position of the new line until both thumbs appear level. Memorise the position of the thumbs. Now cut the new line to the correct position and length. This method can be easily adapted to establish the width of lines and so obtain accurate shapes, even in the most elaborate designs.

Tip

3D effects are produced by the illusion of light and dark within the pattern, representing highlights and shadows. These effects can be created by reducing the thickness of the hair or by leaving the hair longer. The colour of the scalp showing through from beneath helps to create the effect. Remember to establish the position of the light source for highlight and shadow effects (usually from the top of the head) and ensure the effects are created consistently with this light source throughout the design.

The barber must establish the dimensions of the area where the design is to be sited and use scale to design patterns that fit within these dimensions. This can be achieved when using freehand techniques by using estimation and imagining a grid across the area for the design. Features of the object to be replicated are estimated in size and reduced or enlarged to fit within each square of the imaginary grid until the design is complete. The tip on establishing accurate lines can help. But a more scientific method is to produce a stencil, which can be measured accurately and once cut out used to transfer the design accurately to the head.

Proportion

Proportion is similar to scale in that it describes the relative size of one shape or object within a design to the size of another shape or object. It is often referred to by ratios, e.g. we might say that the logo is three times larger than the word in a particular design – a ratio of 3:1. Proportion is important because it helps establish pleasing compositions. The size of the head itself has dimensions that must be considered proportionally within the design, e.g. making the pattern too big may look out of proportion with the size of the head. Proportion establishes whether designs should go over a partial or full head.

Position

Position, or placing, is important to ensure that the pattern is symmetrically placed on the head, unless the design requires an asymmetric design, though here too position is still important. Many factors affect the positioning of patterns in hair, such as hair growth patterns, hair density and proportion. When using freehand techniques the correct position can be established by placing one thumb on the head at arm's length, or by looking in the mirror, and moving the thumb around until it appears to be in the correct place. Stencils may be placed directly on the head and similarly moved around until they appear correct.

Inspiration for the design

Ideas for designs can come from many different sources. Magazines, trade shows and exhibitions are often helpful. Competitions are also good places to see and develop ideas. Popular designs often feature sports and sports clubs or logos and other designs are inspired by events.

Tip

Remember to consider any facial hair in the design of the pattern. The sideburns, moustache, beard and eyebrows can all be features within the design. Complex shapes can be created, but most often it is simple tramlines that are used in facial hair designs.

A 3D pictoral design

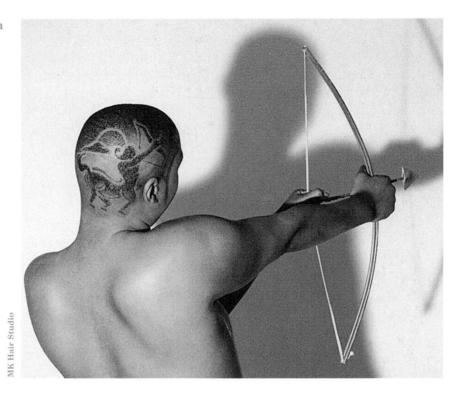

MK Hair Studio

Here are some important things to remember about designing patterns in hair:

- Some patterns are improved by having no distinct outlines. They work best by simply fading out.
- The overall outline of the pattern should usually be cut to appear symmetrical, unless the look is to be asymmetric. Do not just use the ears to determine the position of the pattern, as they are not usually placed level themselves.
- Pay particular attention to where the haircut meets any beard and ensure that they blend together, as required.
- Think of the haircut and moustache and/or beard as being integrated parts of one style.

Cutting techniques

Many cutting techniques, such as scissors-over-comb, clippers-over-comb and freehand are used when creating the foundation haircut for the pattern. These are explained fully in Chapter 5, 'Cutting men's hair using basic techniques'. But there are some techniques that are used especially in creating the pattern itself. These are explained in the following sections.

Channelling

Channelling is the technique used to create complex lines and shapes within the pattern. It is performed with electric clippers or trimmers. The edge of the blades are placed end on to the scalp in order to remove the hair in narrow lines, or placed flat against the scalp to remove hair in the larger shapes. Close cutting fixed blades or the shortest setting on adjustable blades are usually used.

Tramlines or tramlining

Tramlines are a form of channelling where simple lines are created. These are also created with electric clippers or trimmers used with the edge of the blades end on against the scalp.

2D tramline

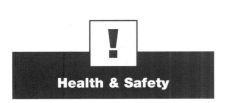

Health & Safety

Great care must be taken when using a razor. Always use light pressure and small movements, as the razor can quickly and easily cut the skin or remove too much hair if not used correctly.

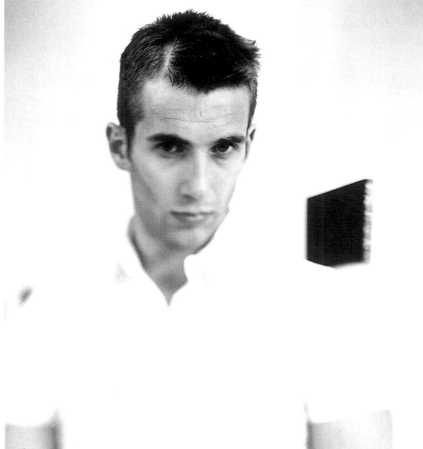

Paul Stafford

Health & Safety

Razors have very sharp blades and must always be treated with care and respect. Keep the handle closed or cover the blade when not in use and especially when carrying or passing them. *Never* place a razor in your pocket and always keep them out of the reach of children.

Razoring

Razoring (shaving) is sometimes used to create cleaner lines and shapes within the pattern. It is performed with a razor, which may be either an open razor or a safety razor. Disposable blade razors are best because they are more hygienic. Electric razors are also sometimes used in larger areas.

Cutting procedures

Many different cutting procedures may be followed to cut men's hair. Individual barbers will usually decide where to start and which cutting techniques to use, mostly according to personal preference. In this work it is the barber's creativity and individualism that comes to the fore. The following examples show how some advanced men's looks can be achieved.

! Health & Safety

Remove excess hair cuttings from the client's face and neck at regular intervals to ensure they are comfortable.

Freehand – 2D graphical pattern

1 Cut the hair to the length required to create a foundation for the pattern.
2 Establish the position of the centre of the pattern on the chosen area of the head.
3 Start in the middle of the pattern and use channelling to outline the first required line or shape according to the chosen scale and proportion.
4 Add additional lines, shapes or extend the single shape, as required working methodically across to one side of the pattern.
5 Return to the centre and repeat step 4 on the other side.
6 Stand back from the client or refer to the mirror regularly to check that the pattern is developing correctly.
7 Remove any unwanted hair from inside the lines, as required.
8 Shave the areas inside the lines if required (see Chapter 11, 'Shaving').

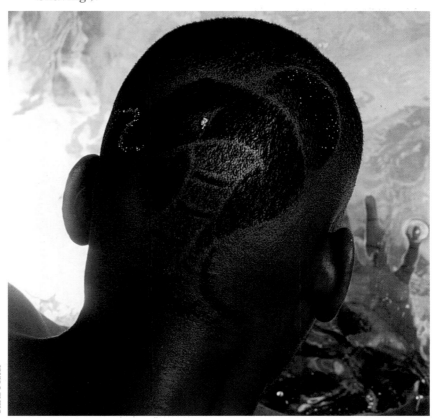

Chris Foster

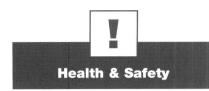

Health & Safety

In this step by step, the stylist uses a razor to complete the design and achieve a close finish. Great care must be taken during this work to avoid causing harm. Use clippers if you are not fully proficient with an open razor. Ensure all areas to be razored are lathered first. See Chapter 11, 'Shaving', for more guidance on shaving around outlines.

2D pictoral pattern

Statue of Liberty

1 Before you begin work on the pattern, cut the area of the hair on which you wish to create a pattern using a number one clipper comb attachment.

2 Now blend the rest of the hair into the cut. This is to make sure that the pattern is clean and fits with the rest of the overall hairstyle.

3 Have your clipper ready to start at the central point on the back of the scalp. This is where the centre of the design will be.

4 When you want to mark straight lines in the pattern you can use your clippers as a basic line guide.

5 If you are not using a stencil refer back to the central point of the design to make sure you are on track.

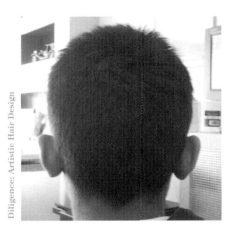

Before cutting

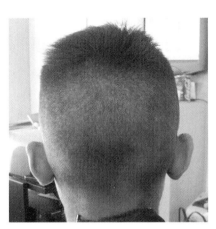

Step 1

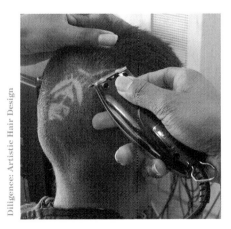

Step 4

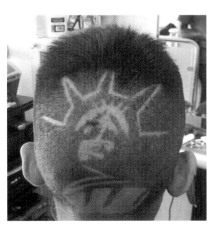

The design begins to emerge

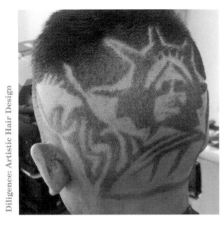

Diligence: Artistic Hair Design

Slide and back view

6 When you have done the central design you can then move onto the parts of the design that are furthest away from the central point. For example, in this step by step the arm of the Statue of Liberty moves away from the central point to the side of the head.

7 When the pattern has been finished you may go on and finish the rest of the cut.

8 Fade the rest of the hair into the design.

9 Shave the areas inside the pattern if necessary (see Chapter 11, 'Shaving').

10 Brush away all the excess hair and brush a light dusting of talcum powder onto the finished cut.

11 Apply gel or wax to finish the cut on the top of the head.

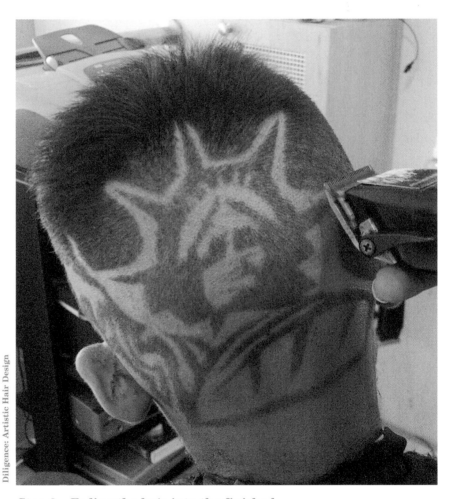

Diligence: Artistic Hair Design

Step 9 – Fading the hair into the finished design

Tip

Cleaner lines and shapes can be achieved by cutting the hair with either close-cutting trimmers or an electric razor. The outline hair may also be removed completely by shaving with a razor, which should be used following the shaving procedure described in Chapter 11, 'Shaving'.

Stencil – 3D pattern

1 Cut the hair to the length required to create a foundation for the pattern.
2 Establish the position of the centre of the pattern on the chosen area of the head and place the centre of the stencil at this point.
3 Adjust the position of the stencil until it appears correct and transfer the design onto the hair by dusting the stencil with a little talc (a light application of hairspray first can help the talc stick to the hair).
4 Start in the middle of the pattern and use channelling to outline the first required line or shape following the marks created by the talc.
5 Add additional lines, shapes or extend the single shape, as required, working methodically across to one side of the pattern.
6 Return to the centre and repeat step 5 on the other side.
7 Stand back from the client or refer to the mirror regularly to check that the pattern is developing correctly.
8 Establish the position of the imagined light source that will be used to produce highlights and shadows within the design.
9 Return to the centre of the pattern and begin removing hair using clippers-over-comb or scissors-over-comb techniques. Try to create the illusion of depth with lighter and darker areas, but remember to keep these consistent with the imagined light source.
10 Remove any unwanted hair from inside the lines, as required.
11 Shave the areas inside the lines if required (see Chapter 11, 'Shaving').

Channelling – a 3D graphical design

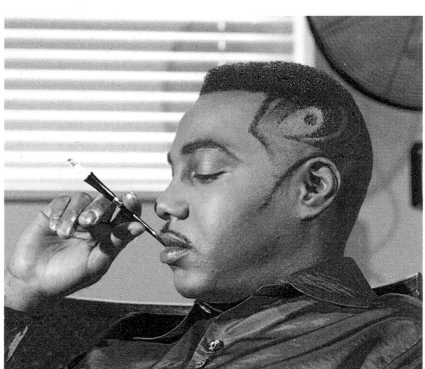

MK Hair Studio

Health and safety

It is important to consider health and safety when creating patterns in hair because of the risks associated with using electricity and the risk of cutting the skin. Here are some important health and safety factors that you must consider when providing hair cutting services:

- If the client has any cuts or abrasions on his face or head, or you suspect that an infection or infestation is present, the work must not be carried out.

- Pay special attention to hygiene when cutting hair because of the risk of cross-infection through open cuts.

- Always protect the client's eyes from hairs with tissues or cotton wool pads when cutting facial hair. Keep your own face away from your work; wear safety glasses for protection.

- Open and safety razors have very sharp blades and must always be handled and used with great care.

- Always close the handle to protect the blade of an open razor when it is not being used or when it is being carried.

- *Never* place razors or other cutting tools in pockets.

- A fixed blade razor must always be *sterilised* before each use.

- A new blade must always be used for each new client when using a detachable blade open razor.

- Used razor blades, called sharps, must be disposed of correctly in accordance with your salon policy. Soiled disposable materials should be placed in sealed plastic bags for removal.

- Electrical equipment must always be handled and used with care in accordance with the manufacturer's instructions.

- *Never* use or place electric clippers or other electrical equipment near water.

- *Do not* go near electrical equipment that is lying in water – isolate the mains power first.

- Visually check that electrical equipment is safe to use before commencing work – check that the cable has not frayed or been pulled and that the plug is not loose.

- Pay attention to the position of cables when using and storing electrical equipment.

- *Never* overload sockets by plugging too many items of electrical equipment into the same socket.

- Follow the manufacturer's instructions for the care of your clippers – ensure that you clean and lubricate the blades regularly to avoid damage.

- Only use clean tools and equipment.

- Make sure that you know the whereabouts of your salon's first-aid kit. Keep yourself up to date with your salon's first-aid and accident procedures.

- Electrical equipment must be regularly tested and given a certificate of testing to confirm that it is safe for use. Your salon owner will ensure that this is carried out, as required.

Activities

1 Visit a library and search the Internet to research ideas for different patterns. Use the information to design pattern stencils that represent different sports, eras, locations, cultures, etc. Your colleagues can then use the stencils in your barber's shop.

2 Take photographs of your best work and produce a style book from the resulting images to help show clients designs they can have. You might also be able to use them to publicise your salon or even to submit them to magazines for wider coverage of your work. Remember to get permission from your manager first.

Check your knowledge

1 Why is it particularly important to accurately establish the type, location and size of pattern to be created?

2 Why is it important to consider hair growth patterns when creating patterns in hair?

3 Why should hair length be considered when cutting hair?

4 Describe the principles of shape and form.

5 Describe how scale is used to decide on the size of pattern to be created.

6 Why can hair density affect the position of a pattern?

7 List three sources of inspiration for hair patterns.

8 Describe how 3D effects are created in a pattern.

9 How can facial hair affect the design of a pattern?

10 Describe the channelling technique.

11 How do tramlines differ from channelling?

12 When might razoring be used to create a pattern?

13 How are stencils used to create patterns?

14 Describe how to maintain high standards of hygiene for using razors.

15 Explain why electrical testing certificates are important.

Index